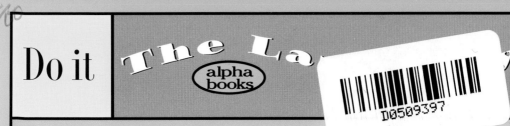

Do it The Lazy Way

D0509397

1. Chunk your workouts. Instead of doing 30 m[inutes at once,] divide your workout into three 10-minute chunks. Pair them with your meals (after breakfast, lunch, and dinner) to spread your calorie burning throughout the day.

2. Don't go all out with your exercise. Just add spurts of effort every now and then to get your body fit and rev up your fat-burning potential. For instance, if you're walking, break into a jog for a little bit.

3. Use your body as resistance for strength training and work several muscle groups at the same time. The more muscles you use, the less time you need to move them.

4. Use items around the house for your strength workout. A few sturdy chairs, some steps (stairway), the kitchen counter, groceries, and water jugs can all be used to build muscles. You can also use your cleaning supplies (broom, duster, mop, vacuum, and so on) to get in a workout while tidying up your house.

5. Strength train in the neighborhood. Use light poles, benches, mailboxes, car bumpers, curbs, and so on to strengthen your muscles outside. Alternate strength exercises with a few minutes of aerobic activity (skipping, walking, step-ups, running, jumping rope) to get a complete workout in one shot.

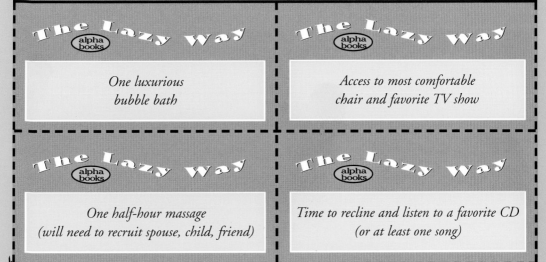

The Lazy Way
alpha books

One luxurious
bubble bath

The Lazy Way
alpha books

Access to most comfortable
chair and favorite TV show

The Lazy Way
alpha books

One half-hour massage
(will need to recruit spouse, child, friend)

The Lazy Way
alpha books

Time to recline and listen to a favorite CD
(or at least one song)

cut

6. Be active during your downtime. Whenever you're waiting for something, get up and move around. If you have to sit for a long period of time, make sure you fidget as much as possible.

7. Wean yourself from technology. Do your daily activities the old-fashioned way: use a manual can opener, rake your leaves, take the stairs, use a wooden spoon, and so on.

8. Size up your portions with your eyes. Keep your meals to no more than two cups of food and don't have more than two to three servings of grains/starches at one meal. Graze on five to six small meals a day.

9. Always carry moisture wipes, a fresh T-shirt, and a pair of sneakers with you. That way, you can work out on the spot and clean up in a jiffy.

10. Create a monthly progress report (see Chapter 4) to track your exercise, eating, and attitude. It will just take a few minutes each day to log your workouts, and at the end of the month, you can see your progress at a glance.

The Lazy Way

alpha books

COUPON

The Lazy Way

alpha books

COUPON

The Lazy Way

alpha books

COUPON

The Lazy Way

alpha books

COUPON

cut

Get in
Shape

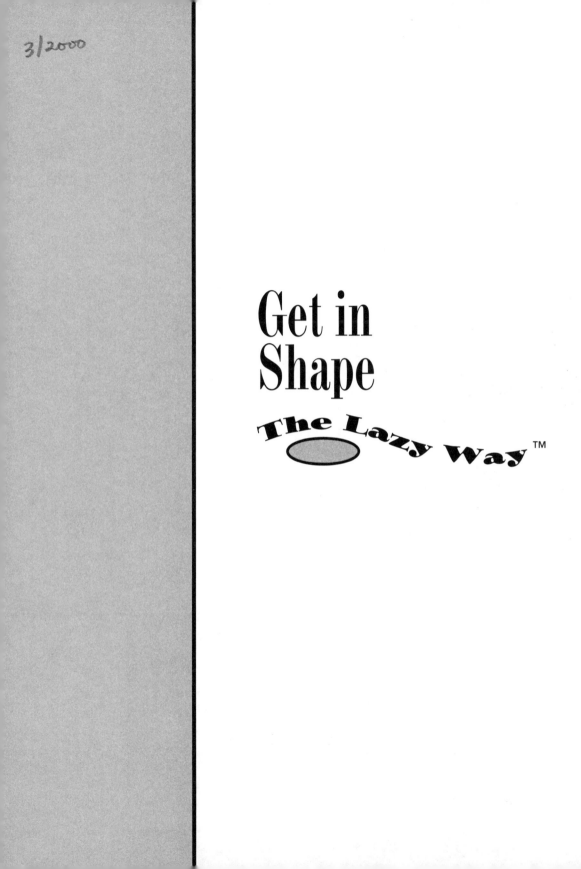

The Lazy Way™

Get in Shape

Annette Cain

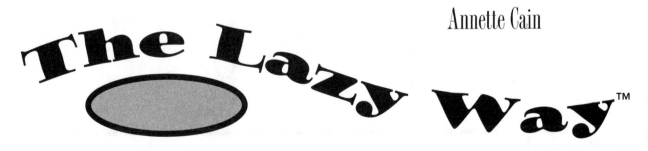

Macmillan • USA

To my parents, with deep gratitude, for shaping me up with their unconditional love and support.

Macmillan Publishing books may be purchased for business or sales promotional use. For information please write: Special Markets Department, Macmillan Publishing USA, 1633 Broadway, New York, NY 10019.

International Standard Book Number: 0-02-863010-6
Library of Congress Catalog Card Number: 98-89559

00 99   8   7   6   5   4   3   2   1

Interpretation of the printing code: the rightmost number of the first series of numbers is the year of the book's printing; the rightmost number of the second series of numbers is the number of the book's printing. For example, a printing code of 99-1 shows that the first printing occurred in 1999.

Printed in the United States of America

Book Design: Madhouse Studios

Page Creation: Carrie Allen and Heather Pope

You Don't Have to Feel Guilty Anymore!

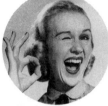

IT'S O.K. TO DO IT *THE LAZY WAY*!

It seems every time we turn around, we're given more responsibility, more information to absorb, more places we need to go, and more numbers, dates, and names to remember. Both our bodies and our minds are already on overload. And we know what happens next—cleaning the house, balancing the checkbook, and cooking dinner get put off until "tomorrow" and eventually fall by the wayside.

So let's be frank—we're all starting to feel a bit guilty about the dirty laundry, stacks of ATM slips, and Chinese takeout. Just thinking about tackling those terrible tasks makes you exhausted, right? If only there were an easy, effortless way to get this stuff done! (And done right!)

There is—*The Lazy Way*! By providing the pain-free way to do something—including tons of shortcuts and timesaving tips, as well as lists of all the stuff you'll ever need to get it done efficiently—*The Lazy Way* series cuts through all of the time-wasting thought processes and laborious exercises. You'll discover the secrets of those who have figured out *The Lazy Way*. You'll get things done in half the time it takes the average person—and then you will sit back and smugly consider those poor suckers who haven't discovered *The Lazy Way* yet. With *The Lazy Way,* you'll learn how to put in minimal effort and get maximum results so you can devote your attention and energy to the pleasures in life!

v

THE LAZY WAY PROMISE

Everyone on *The Lazy Way* staff promises that, if you adopt *The Lazy Way* philosophy, you'll never break a sweat, you'll barely lift a finger, you won't put strain on your brain, and you'll have plenty of time to put up your feet. We guarantee you will find that these activities are no longer hardships, since you're doing them *The Lazy Way*. We also firmly support taking breaks and encourage rewarding yourself (we even offer our suggestions in each book!). With *The Lazy Way*, the only thing you'll be overwhelmed by is all of your newfound free time!

THE LAZY WAY SPECIAL FEATURES

Every book in our series features the following sidebars in the margins, all designed to save you time and aggravation down the road.

- **"Quick 'n' Painless"**—shortcuts that get the job done fast.
- **"You'll Thank Yourself Later"**—advice that saves time down the road.
- **"A Complete Waste of Time"**—warnings that spare countless headaches and squandered hours.
- **"If You're So Inclined"**—optional tips for moments of inspired added effort.
- **"The Lazy Way"**—rewards to make the task more pleasurable.

If you've either decided to give up altogether or have taken a strong interest in the subject, you'll find information on hiring outside help with "How to Get Someone Else to Do It" as well as further reading recommendations in "If You Really Want More, Read These." In addition, there's an only-what-you-need-to-know glossary of terms and product names ("If You Don't Know What It Means/Does, Look Here") as well as "It's Time for Your Reward"—fun and relaxing ways to treat yourself for a job well done.

With *The Lazy Way* series, you'll find that getting the job done has never been so painless!

Series Editor
Amy Gordon

Cover Designer
Michael Freeland

Editorial Director
Gary Krebs

Managing Editor
Robert Shuman

Director of Creative Services
Michele Laseau

Development Editor
Alana Morgan

Production Editor
Carol Sheehan

What's in This Book

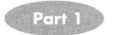
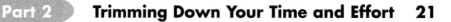

Don't Sweat It!

Does sweat bead off your forehead with the mere thought of getting in shape? The pain and strain of countless reps and sets, constricting clothes, complicated formulas, and convoluted equipment is bound to leave you wringing wet.

Ditch the drudgery and get in shape *The Lazy Way!* You can stay fit without a daily grind on your body or your schedule. Toning up *The Lazy Way* is all about:

- Trimming down your time and effort
- Working out in the comfort of your own home
- Furnishing your own fitness supplies from cupboards and closets
- Using what you've got, on the spot
- Tuning into the bare minimum level you need to work at to get results
- Getting your muscles firm, without the squirm
- Loosening up your body from the pressures of the workday
- Having some time to relax

So follow the practically effortless plan in this book and ease yourself into shape!

THANK YOU...

To my beloved hubby, Greg, for putting up with cereal for dinner on more than a few occasions! Thanks, sweetie, for keeping me sane and smiling.

To my agent, Martha Casselman, who always gives her best swing when she's at bat for me.

To Jim Vaughn who never complained about my chicken scratches and was there every single time I needed him.

To my good girlfriend and great physical therapist, Lauri Merrill, who always keeps me straight with my exercise descriptions.

To Vern Gambetta and Gary Gray for their ingenious 3 x 3 x 3 matrix—it's the best use for a pair of dumbbells that I've ever seen!

To everyone at San Tomo for letting me step on their toes. Joan and Dino, thanks for everything (I mean everything!).

To Alana Morgan and the team at Macmillan for shaping up my sentences.

Disclaimer

This book is not intended as a substitute for professional medical advice. As with all exercise programs, you should get your physician's approval before beginning this program, especially if you have a medical problem such as diabetes, high blood pressure, or heart disease. The author disclaims any liability arising directly or indirectly from the use and application of any of the contents of this book.

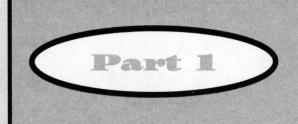

Part 1

Simply Sizing Up Your Needs

Are You Too Lazy to Read Simply Sizing Up Your Needs?

1 Your stationary bike has more clothes on it than you do. ☐ yes ☐ no

2 You think a leotard should be an endangered species. ☐ yes ☐ no

3 Your definition of a dumbbell is someone who pumps iron. ☐ yes ☐ no

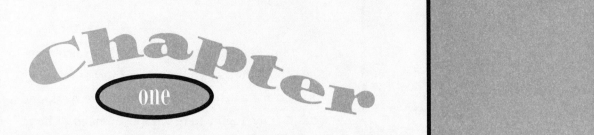

Chapter one

Don't Be a Dumbbell!

It starts with the New Year's resolution to get in shape. Immediately, the vicious exercise cycle of too much, too hard, too soon begins, leaving you too dead to keep it up. After awhile you figure the best thing to do is rest and recuperate until the following year. Sound familiar?

For some reason, most of us think we have to torture ourselves into shape. Maybe it's because we've too often heard, "No pain, no gain!" or "Go for the burn!" Fortunately, getting fit doesn't have to make you feel as though you checked yourself into boot camp.

In this chapter, I'll show you how to leave the torment behind. You'll discover all the things you don't have to do, along with what you need to know to get in shape *The Lazy Way.* You'd be a dumbbell to do it any other way.

FORGET THE FANCY FORMULAS

The first thing you don't have to do is worry about calculating frequency multiplied by duration multiplied by intensity or any other unnecessary fitness formulas. The only thing that's necessary is to do the exercise—*The Lazy Way,* of course.

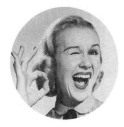

- You don't need heart rate monitors or calculators to figure out whether you're in your target zone. If you become a little heated, a little breathless, and a little sweaty, then you're where you need to be to get results. (Turn to Chapter 6 for more details on your heart rate zone.)

- Don't give yourself a hernia trying to determine what your maximum rep is (the heaviest amount of weight you can lift once). You don't have to lift a certain percentage of your maximum rep to see a difference in your muscles. (Chapters 10, 11, and 12 show you how you can build up your muscles without breaking down.)

- You don't have to lift so many sets of so many repetitions either. I'll explain how to do just the right amount to strengthen and tone your muscles.

- You've probably heard that you need to do at least 20 minutes of aerobic activity at least four times a week. This guideline doesn't mean that you have to cramp your schedule with big blocks of workout time. You can reap the health benefits without the time constraints. A few minutes of exercise here and there will do the trick, too.

- Speaking of numbers, forget about your bathroom scale. Usually, when you want to get in shape, you also want to lose some pounds. Think in terms of losing inches instead. That way, when you gain some muscle weight, you won't get discouraged.

FREE YOURSELF FROM THE IRON BARS OF THE GYM

You may think you need to put in some mandatory gym time to get results. So you join the local health club, but as time goes by, the only thing that gets trim is your wallet. It's time to break free from the notion that you need fancy equipment or long hours at the gym to get in shape. You can always work out on the spot with what you've got.

- You can get a complete strength workout in the comfort of your own home. Whether you're in the shower, at the kitchen sink, or on the couch, strength training at home has never been more simple and effective.

- You can fit in some easy exercises during your down time at the office. Waiting while on the phone, sending a fax, or making copies are perfect opportunities to get physical.

- Take advantage of the time you spend on the road. Getting fit while you sit is one of the secrets to shaping up *The Lazy Way*. Chapter 9 will give you a trunkful of tips to tone you up behind the wheel.

- Your body is the best resistance machine ever made, which makes it the prime choice when choosing your equipment. Turn to Chapter 10 to discover several easy ways you can prod your bod.

- You don't have to waste your money on fancy gadgets to get you fit. You can make your own dumbbells from household containers.

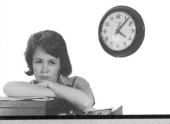

A COMPLETE WASTE OF TIME

The 3 Worst Things to Do at the Gym:

1. Sign up for an annual membership.

2. Get stuck in the fitness equipment.

3. Drop a dumbbell on your toe.

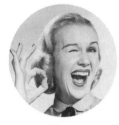

GIVE YOURSELF A BACKBONE SO YOU WON'T BACK OUT

If you want to stay fit for the rest of your life, you need to exercise for the rest of your life (scary thought!). Here are some tips to help lessen the chill and double the thrill of this lifelong process:

- Pick activities you enjoy. If you don't particularly find any part of exercise pleasurable, add certain elements (music, nature, friends) to make it more enjoyable.

- Choose a variety of aerobic activities and a good mix of resistance and flexibility exercises. This variety will help enhance your overall fitness and keep you from boredom and injury.

- Give yourself some fitness goals to strive for. Realistic goals not only motivate you, but they also give you a sense of accomplishment when you achieve them.

- Find a workout buddy. Your chances of staying with your exercise program are greatly enhanced when you have a friend to work out with.

- Make your fitness regimen as convenient as possible. It has to be hassle-free, or you're not going to stick with it. Lucky for you, shaping up *The Lazy Way* is all about convenience.

BECOME A MUSCLE BUFF, NOT A MUSCLE HEAD

The thought of gaining muscle can weigh heavily on the mind. You may shy away from strength training because you are fearful of looking too much like Arnold or tipping the bathroom scale. But muscle is your friend, and here are some reasons why you should be its biggest fan.

- Strength training *The Lazy Way* is not going to give you bulging muscles, but it will increase your muscle mass. This is a good thing because the more muscle you have, the more fat you will burn.

- Stronger muscles yield stronger bones. You'll slow down the loss of function associated with aging and reduce the possibility of muscle and tendon injuries.

- Strength training increases your mobility and coordination and improves your balance and stability.

- Proper strength exercise helps you maintain proper body posture and protects against lower back injury. See Chapters 10 through 13 for descriptions of several simple exercises.

- Getting stronger enhances your ability to perform daily physical tasks without injury or discomfort.

SOLVE THE RIDDLE OF LOSING FAT AROUND YOUR MIDDLE

Somewhere along the line, we've been led to think that doing sit-ups will get rid of the flab around our middles. That's a bunch of "pork-belly wash"! Here are some answers to the riddle of losing fat around your middle:

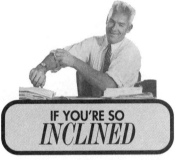

IF YOU'RE SO INCLINED

You can make the most of your downtime at work if you keep a couple of small weights in your desk drawer. The next time you're waiting for a fax or printout, pick up the weights for an extra boost.

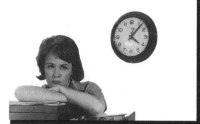

If you are carrying fat around your middle, the best way to get rid of it is with aerobic exercise, not stomach crunches.

Forget about doing 300 sit-ups. You can strengthen and tone your abdominals with just a few simple exercises. (Check out Chapter 13 for more details.)

Yes, there is such a thing as 'middle-age spread,' especially if you are a woman with wacky hormones. Don't beat yourself up about it, just pound those fat cells out of you with some aerobic exercise. It's your best defense.

If you are carrying more weight around your middle, you may be putting yourself at risk for heart disease. You can find out if you are at risk by measuring your waist to hip ratio. Divide your waist measurement by your hip measurement. Ideally, women should have a waist/hip ratio of 0.8 or less, and men should have 0.9 or less.

Here's a cruel weight loss fact: The last place you see fat go is where you have it the most. This is why it might take you longer to see your belly disappear. Just be patient and stick to the Lazy shape-up rules. You'll whittle your waist down without any side aches.

Shaping up *The Lazy Way* does not involve figuring out calculations, fumbling with equipment, or taking up all your free time. You'll have everything to gain with none of the pain. Granted, you're not going to look like a supermodel or Greek statue, but you will definitely become more fit and toned.

Getting Time on Your Side

	The Old Way	The Lazy Way
Calculating fitness formulas	30 minutes	0 minutes
Getting in your workout	At least 45 minutes	A few minutes, here and there
Doing sit-ups	10 minutes	2 to 5 minutes
Getting ready to work out	20 minutes	2 seconds
Achieving your goals	Maybe never	You're on the home stretch!
Feeling good when you work out	Is it possible?	This feels great!

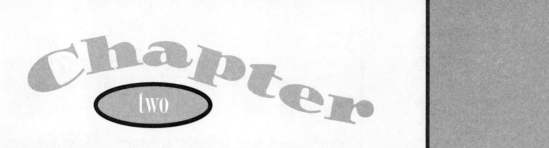

Left to Your Own Devices

If only fitness equipment could talk. Hundreds, no, thousands of exercise gadgets and gizmos would reveal horrific tales of abuse and neglect. From the very beginning, their worth was undercut with "three easy payments." Then they were shoved in a corner and suffocated by dust or clothes, only to be undersold once again in a garage sale. And to think, all they longed for was to be coated with a little warmth and sweat.

For some reason, we think having a machine at home will give us the results that its infomercial boldly promises. It never seems to work out that way, which is just as well, because who needs to spend precious time and money on things that will just clutter up the house? The key is to keep your fitness equipment simple. Use what you have around you, such as a chair, a step, or your own body (that's down-to-the-bones simple!).

You're left to your own devices when you get in shape *The Lazy Way.* In this chapter, I'll show you how to furnish your own fitness supplies from things around your house and make

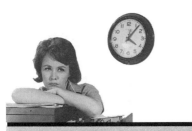

the most of what your neighborhood has to offer. I'll also give you tips on choosing a personal trainer and gearing yourself up to go.

FEELING RIGHT AT HOME IN YOUR HOMEMADE GYM

When it comes to shaping up, you want to go for comfort, celerity, and convenience. And what could be more comfy and speedy than working out at home? Plus, there's nothing more handy than using some of the items around your house to get the calories stirring. So pull up a sofa, and let's get ready to tumble!

Poof! Instant Fitness Equipment Under Your Roof

You don't have to look far for these sturdy pieces of equipment. They're right under your roof:

- A bench
- Kitchen counter
- A heavy block of wood (you may have to look in your garage for this one)
- A sturdy table
- Stairway/steps
- Two sturdy chairs

Hold the Bells and Whistles

Remember, you don't need anything fancy when it comes to working out. You can find most of the items you need right around the house. You can buy other fitness tools at your local sports store or order them from the catalogs listed in the back of this book.

These simple supplies will do the trick, depending on which activity you pick:

- Birdseed
- Broom
- Buckshot
- Clock (or watch with second hand)
- Dumbbells (two each of 2 pounds, 5 pounds, 8 pounds, 10 pounds, 15 pounds)
- Exercise balls
- Gallon jugs
- Jump rope
- Mat
- Mop
- Music (stereo or portable cassette/CD player)
- Pool accessories (noodles, aqua gloves, foam dumbbells)
- Sand
- Scale
- Soup cans
- Surgical tubing or rubber exercise bands (cut into four-foot strips)
- Water bottles
- Weighted wrist bands
- Workout videos

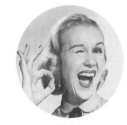

QUICK ⬤ PAINLESS

The kitchen sink is not just for washing dishes. You can use it for squats, dips, and presses, too. Make sure your hands aren't soapy, though.

Here's a simple recipe for making your own home-made dumbbells:

1. Gather some empty plastic containers from around the house. They can be gallon jugs (for milk, bleach, and so on) or smaller water bottles.

2. Fill the containers with sand, birdseed, or buckshot (you can find the latter at your local hardware or hunting store). These fillers are listed in weight from lightest to heaviest.

3. Weigh each container on a scale to create a set of 2-pound, 5-pound, 8-pound, and 10-pound weights (two of each).

4. Label each container with the appropriate weight.

Plotting Your Progress

You need to gather a few supplies to help you keep track of your gains (strength, goals, and so on) and your losses (inches, pounds, and so on):

- Aerobic training log
- Calendar
- Event calendars (from local paper or fitness magazine)
- Journal
- Measurement record
- Daily planner
- Post-It Notes
- Strength training log

IF YOU'RE SO
INCLINED

You can make your own homemade dumbbells with empty water bottles or milk jugs and some sand or birdseed. If you want to make Martha Stewart proud, add some tassels or a monogram.

IT'S A BEAUTIFUL DAY IN THE NEIGHBORHOOD

There's no place like home, but it's not the only place where you can get in shape. Your neighborhood has a lot to offer, too. Whether it's a nearby park, the city recreation department, or a local health club, there are many avenues you can choose to get fit. In this book, I'll show you what to take advantage of in your neighborhood and how not to be taken advantage of by health clubs.

Let Your Surroundings Stir You

Your aerobic and strength conditioning can be a walk in the park (or a jaunt down the street)! The key is to incorporate your surroundings into your workout. Here are a few environmental props you can lean on for support:

- Benches
- Curbs
- Mailboxes
- Golf courses
- Parks/green belts
- Playground equipment
- Streetlights

Looking for Movement in All the Right Places

Your community has a vast array of activities that you can choose from depending on what you fancy. One of the best ways to discover what's out there is to sit down with the phone book (be sure to put your feet up!) and thumb

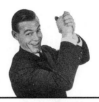

Keep track of the number of repetitions and/or the amount of weight you lift when strength training. That way you'll be able to see how much stronger you become over time.

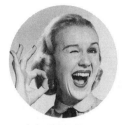

QUICK ◼ PAINLESS

through the pages. Check out the following resources to help point you in the right direction:

- Activity clubs in the community (such as walking, hiking, or biking clubs)
- Adult education programs
- City recreation department
- Company fitness center
- Dance studios
- Health clubs
- Jazzercise studios
- Junior college physical education classes
- Karate classes
- Malls (walking groups)
- Masters swimming programs
- Pilatus studios
- YMCA or YWCA
- Yoga centers

Don't Get Aced by Clubs

If you are willing to put up with the inconvenience of traveling to your workout, then you may want to look into joining a local health club. But sometimes the chrome jungle, high-paced classes, and loud grunts can be a little intimidating. (Who needs to get all worked up before they even work out?) There's no need to worry because you're not like everyone else who joins a club to get their hearts (and other body parts) in shape. You will have a card up your sleeve—you'll know how to get in shape *The Lazy Way.*

Use these tips to keep your club workout simple and anxiety-free:

- Find out what the quietest hours of the club are and plan to go there during those times. You'll be able to zip in and out when fewer people are around.

- Make an appointment with a qualified trainer or instructor to help you design a program specifically for you. Most clubs usually offer a free fitness evaluation or session with an in-house instructor.

- You can do any of the simple exercises described in Chapters 10 through 12 and get a complete strength workout without getting tangled up in the machines at the club. Sticking to free weights is your best bet, and most clubs have more dumbbells than they can handle.

- You can usually choose from a variety of classes. Go for the beginner ones that keep the pace slower, and be sure to work out at a level that's comfortable for you.

- Instead of torturing yourself with lots of grueling minutes on one machine, pick three or four different machines and alternate them. Stay just long enough to warm the seat, and then move on to the next one.

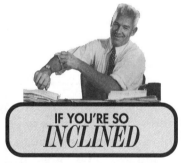

IF YOU'RE SO
INCLINED

Next time you're shopping at the mall, find out if it opens early for walking groups. This is a great way to take your walking indoors when the weather gets bad.

HOUSE CALLS MAY PREVENT SERIOUS FALLS

If you find that you need a gentle push to help you get off your tush, then consider hiring a personal trainer. These fitness professionals come in all shapes and sizes, but what's important is their style. Here are some criteria for choosing trainers that will help you get in shape *The Lazy Way:*

1. They are willing to come to your house.

2. They highly recommend this book.

3. They've never owned, borrowed, or used a whip.

Another important thing is that they must know what they are talking about. Make sure your prospective trainer is currently certified. These are the best-known, most recognizable certifying organizations:

■ Aerobics and Fitness Association of America (AFAA)

■ American Council on Exercise (ACE)

■ American College of Sports Medicine (ACSM)

■ National Academy of Sports Medicine (NASM)

■ National Strength and Conditioning Association (NSCA)

■ The Cooper Clinic

You can find personal trainers through health clubs, hospitals, and/or physical therapy clinics. Be sure to request references so that you can ask their clients if they think the trainer is getting them in shape *The Lazy Way.*

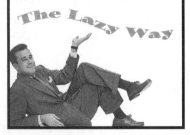

Congratulations! You've found yourself a personal trainer to keep you going when you need it most! Now get yourself to the nearest park and enjoy some fresh air!

The Lazy Way

MOVING COMFORTS

Some of today's fitness apparel is easy on the eyes, especially when it's on somebody else. You definitely want to stay away from anything that gives you a workout just trying to put it on. Your best bet is to stick with loose, breathable, comfy outfits that you could sleep in if you needed to. Add a few other necessary items to keep you fresh and dry, and you've geared yourself to go.

Here are some comforts you wouldn't want to move without:

- Deodorant
- Fresh undies
- Moisture wipes
- Sneakers
- Sweat bands
- Towel(s)
- Water bottle
- Workout bag
- Workout clothes (T-shirt, shorts, socks)

When you're left to your own devices you can work out whenever, wherever, and with whomever you want. You make the rules. Whatever helps you exercise regularly is the right thing for you.

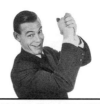

YOU'LL THANK YOURSELF LATER

Keep a clean set of undies along with your toiletries in your workout bag, just in case you happen to sweat too much.

Getting Time on Your Side

	The Old Way	The Lazy Way
Working out at home	1 hour	10 to 30 minutes
Working out in the neighborhood	1 hour	10 to 30 minutes
Working out at the club	$1\frac{1}{2}$ hours	10 to 30 minutes
Working out with a trainer	1 hour	30 minutes max!
Getting your equipment ready to work out	5 to 7 minutes	0 to 2 minutes
Getting you ready to work out	15 minutes	3 to 5 minutes

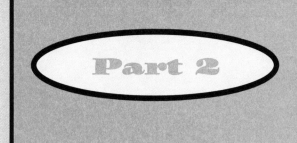

Trimming Down Your Time and Effort

Are You Too Lazy to Read Trimming Down Your Time and Effort?

1 You haven't gotten rid of your love handles because you think they make you more romantic. ☐ yes ☐ no

2 Your favorite exercise routine is watching *ESPN*. ☐ yes ☐ no

3 The thought of getting sweaty makes you break out in hives. ☐ yes ☐ no

Defining the Details

Getting in shape *The Lazy Way* is a lot like carving a statue. You start with a lump of putty, and then, little by little, you slowly transform it into a solid figure with lots of smooth curves and fine lines. But the true masterpiece is achieved only after you define the details.

This isn't as tedious as it sounds. Defining the details just means focusing on the things that are the most important for molding you into shape with the least amount of effort. Such details include getting time on your side, choosing activities you enjoy, setting realistic goals, tracking your progress, and shaping up your diet. When you define these details ahead of time you save yourself a lot of wasted energy (just ask Michelangelo!). So roll up your sleeves and get ready to chisel away, and you'll be able to unveil yourself with pride. It may take a little time, but you're worth it!

TIME IS ON YOUR SIDE

Even though it takes some time to see results, you don't have to spend all your time trying to get them. All you need is a mere 30 minutes a day, and you don't even have to rack up those minutes all at once! You can do a little here and a little there, whatever your heart, legs, and lungs desire.

These tips will help you get time on your side (and as time goes by, you'll have less on your sides):

- The first thing you should do is plan your day of rest. Pick the day of the week that you are the busiest or the laziest. On this day, you have my permission to refrain from lifting a finger (even your pinky).

- It's a good rule to take only one rest day at a time. Don't go more than one day without lifting a finger.

- The time of the day you exercise doesn't matter much. What matters is that you fit in your workout time when it's the most convenient for you.

- Forget about trying to get in at least 30 minutes of exercise at a time. You can get the same benefits by breaking this 30-minute chunk into three smaller, 10-minute nuggets. You'll find that whittling down your workouts is much easier on your schedule.

- Spend a few minutes each week scheduling your exercise time in your planner or day calendar. Slip these appointments in wherever they are the most convenient.

YOU CAN'T LOSE WHEN YOU GET TO CHOOSE

Your exercise needs to be enjoyable, or you won't stick with it long enough to get in shape. Luckily, there are

Congratulations! You decided to schedule your exercise time. The first thing you should do is plan your day of rest. (That's an order from higher sources!)

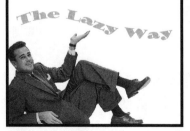

The Lazy Way

lots of ways to find pleasure working out. Bringing a friend along, being outdoors, and listening to music are just a few elements that add to the fun. Decide what makes exercise enjoyable for you, because there's nothing to lose (except for pounds and inches!) when you get to choose!

The following elements will give your workouts ever-ready, long-lasting power—you'll keep going and going and going!

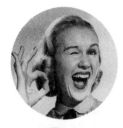

QUICK ⬭ *PAINLESS*

Think of your workouts as important appointments to keep with yourself. When you make a doctor or dentist appointment, you know the date and time, and you're there! That's how it should be with your workouts, too.

- Make your exercise playful. Remember how much fun it was playing when you were a kid? You don't have to stop having fun now that you're all grown up. Think of activities and games that you enjoyed participating in and start playing them again.

- Use the seasons to guide you to new exercise experiences. Each season offers different recreational activities. For instance, in the spring, you might hike to see the wildflowers; in the summer, you may hang out in the water; in autumn, you could ride your bike amidst the fall foliage; and in winter, you may want to have some fun in the snow.

- Choose a buddy to work out with. This is one of the best ways to ensure that you will get the most enjoyment and longevity with your exercise program.

- Sometimes it's a matter of choosing an exercise that's most convenient when it comes to finding an activity that works best for you. Walking probably fits the bill for most. After all, you carry your legs with you wherever you go. All you need to do is add some sneakers, and you're off!

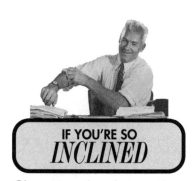

Choose a cleaning-up-the-house day as one of your workouts for the week. You may get a little dirty and sweaty, but your house will get sparkling clean.

░ You are the boss of your exercise routine. So you have the power to manage it any way you please. For instance, you may decide to institute a work-around-the-house day. Not only does this day relieve you from the normal exercise routine, it also allows you to burn some calories and clean your house at the same time.

AIM FOR THE SKIES, AND YOU'LL MELT YOUR THUNDER THIGHS

You won't get far if you don't have goals. Of course, you won't get very far if you have unrealistic goals either. How can you aim for the skies without turning your dreams into lies? Just follow these guidelines, and you'll be soaring in no time:

░ Keep your goals realistic! You'll probably never swim the English Channel if you're afraid you might drown in the bathtub. When setting your goals, don't set yourself up for failure. Know what your limits are and only set goals that are real for you.

░ Keep your goals short-term! I know what you're thinking. You want to get in shape overnight—you can't get more short-term than that, right? Of course, you and I both know that the only way we could shape up overnight is with an airbrush. Because getting in shape is a lengthy process, having short-term goals will get you to the end result a lot quicker.

░ Keep your goals specific! Don't settle for general statements such as, "I want to get in shape." What is it about your shape that you want to change (without having to go to a body parts store)? Do you want to lose some weight? How many pounds? Do you want to tone your muscles? All of them or just your calves?

- Keep your goals flexible! You can't blame yourself if you wanted to ski last winter, but it didn't snow. Your goals need to be as flexible as the weather. If you keep them too rigid, they're bound to freeze you up over time.

- Keep your goals action-oriented! It's easy to get caught up in how you want to be, rather than what you will do to get there. Keep your focus on the doing and that will create your being.

- Last, but not least, reward yourself for achieving your goals. Of course, you will already be feeling the warm glow that comes with accomplishment, but you deserve more. Have a list of rewards or treats that you can choose from every time you achieve one of your goals.

DON'T BE A LUMP ON THE LOG

Keeping an exercise log can be a drag if it's a cross to bear. The key is to not make it a big ordeal. Focus on the elements that have the most weight, such as minutes spent exercising, repetitions lifted, or inches lost. Spending a little time keeping track of a few fundamentals will be a pleasure instead of a burden.

Take note of these tips for successful logging:

Congratulations! You achieved one of your goals! Now it's time to celebrate. Take out your reward list, and choose a prize that will make you feel special.

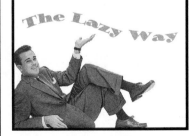

The Lazy Way

Schedule your measurement days (every six weeks) into your day calendar. Time flies when you're having fun, so planning these dates in advance will keep you from skipping your measurement days.

- You will notice measurable changes in your body's shape every four to six weeks. Plan to weigh and measure yourself at six-week intervals. Take some time to schedule these measurement dates in your planner.

- When you keep track of the weights or repetitions you are lifting, you will be able to see yourself growing stronger from one week to the next.

- Log the minutes you spend doing aerobic activities so that you can behold how the little nuggets add up to a big chunk of time. You'll be surprised at how quickly a few minutes here and there will accumulate.

- The number of calories burned is a good thing to keep track of, especially if you want to observe your caloric deficit in action. You want to burn around 1500 to 2000 calories with your weekly physical activity. The caloric chart in Chapter 7 can help you determine the number of calories you burn from exercise.

- Whenever you try a new activity, you might want to jot down how the experience was. Did you like it? Do you want to keep it on your list? Or do you never want to be there and do that again? If you needed to use special equipment, write down a few details about the equipment (sizes, brands, and so on) so that you can refer to them the next time you want to do the activity.

- If you find an activity to be less than fun, take some time to see how you can make it better, before giving up on it. You may find that all you need is a little music or a buddy to turn the experience around for you!

- Take a moment to note your energy level. Do you feel rested when you get up in the morning? Are you dragging by mid-afternoon? Do you feel more tired after exercising, instead of being energized? Observing your energy level can help you discern whether you're over-loaded.

A MOMENT ON YOUR LIPS DOESN'T HAVE TO MEAN A LIFETIME ON YOUR HIPS

You can subtract a lot of calories with your workouts, but you can't forget how they add up with your eating. If you are serious about shaping up your body, then you have to shape up your eating habits as well. Don't worry; you don't need to go on a diet! A trim here and a shave there can do the trick.

Pile on these nuggets, and you'll shape up your plate:

- Eat a variety of wholesome foods. This variety will provide you with a diet of mostly complex carbohy-drates (including fruits and vegetables), moderate amounts of protein, small amounts of fat and sweets, and lots of fiber, vitamins, and minerals.

- Be sure to get in plenty of water. Drink at least 64 ounces throughout the day. If you tend to sweat a lot, you can end up losing a bunch of water. A pound of weight lost during exercise is equivalent to losing two cups of water. Weigh yourself before and

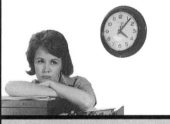

A COMPLETE WASTE OF TIME

The 3 Worst Ways to Shape Up Your Diet:

1. Guzzling raw eggs. (Rocky may have done this, but he was hit in the head a lot, too!)

2. Giving up chocolate.

3. Wiring your jaw shut.

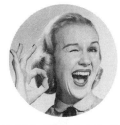

after exercise and drink two cups of water for every pound lost.

- You don't want to be starving before your workouts. If you haven't eaten for more than three or four hours, you probably won't have much energy when you exercise. Keep some wholesome snacks handy for times when you need an energy boost.

- Take a multivitamin/mineral supplement to enhance your diet. Don't buy anything fancy, just make sure it has no more than 150 percent of the RDA, no fillers, and no artificial colors.

- Never let yourself get hungry or full. Aim for five to six small meals throughout the day.

- If you want to shed some pounds, you can't do it by exercise alone. You also need to cut back on what you eat. Eating a little less combined with your activity will create a healthy caloric deficit. You need to be in a deficit of 3500 calories to lose one pound of body fat.

- Forget about dieting; it just doesn't work! There is no magic food or supplement that's going to melt off your fat. The best way to shape up your diet is to follow the tips presented here along with the shortcuts in the next chapter.

Getting Time on Your Side

	The Old Way	The Lazy Way
Planning your exercise time	15 minutes	5 minutes
Tracking your progress	10 minutes	5 minutes
Choosing your activities	5 minutes	1 minute
Setting your goals	Hours	Minutes
Achieving your goals	Never	Always
Shaping up your diet	Months	Days

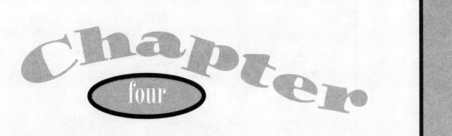

Chapter four

In a Pinch

It's not that you don't want to get in shape. It's just a little hard for you to fathom how you can fit one more thing into your schedule. But you want to fit into your jeans, so you figure it's worth the struggle. Let me assure you that it doesn't have to be a tight squeeze.

Your shape-up tasks will not be binding if you take a few shortcuts. In this chapter, you'll discover all sorts of ways to shorten your workout time, cut back on your eating, and quickly track your progress. So jump into those cutoffs and breathe a sigh of relief.

WHIZ THROUGH YOUR WORKOUTS

As mentioned before, you can whiz through your workouts if you break your 30-minute block of exercise time into smaller chunks, but this is just one of the ways to get fit. Follow these tips, and you'll get through your workout in no time:

- Plan your exercise time first thing in the morning (especially when everyone's still sleeping). Exercising in the morning means minimum interruptions and maximum energy for your day.

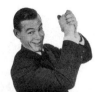

- Pair your 10-minute chunks of exercise with your meals. You can do them before or after your breakfast, lunch, and dinner. Either way, following this schedule spreads your calorie-burning activity throughout the day.

- If you don't have 10 minutes to spare, you can divvy your workouts into even smaller chunks. Plan on doing six-minute chunks of exercise with your regular meals and after your mid-morning and afternoon snacks.

- On days when your schedule is too full for a 30-minute session, you can still shape up by taking advantage of your down time (for example, waiting on the phone, sending a fax, or making copies). Check out the fitness tips in Chapter 9 for ideas on how to make the most of your down time. That way, you can whiz through your workouts no matter how demanding your day is.

- You can work out on the spot when you wear your tennis shoes to work (or keep them nearby). Then all you have to do is grab your legs and go.

WEIGHTS WITH NO WAITING

You may think strength training will take up a load of your time, especially if you do it at the gym, but you can whiz right through your weight workouts too. These simple and savvy shortcuts will keep you from waiting when working with weights:

- Don't waste your time lifting weights for separate muscles when you can work several muscles with one movement. For instance, instead of doing bicep curls and then tricep extensions, do some push-ups or dips. These multimuscle moves not only work your arms but your chest and back, too.

- As long as you're working more than one muscle at a time, you can be even more efficient and combine upper and lower body movements. For example, do lunges with your legs and curls with your arms at the same time. (You might not want to chew gum with this one!)

- You deserve a break after lifting a set, but if you want to save time, do back-to-back sets that work opposing muscle groups. So if you just finished a set of dumbbell presses (chest) you can go right into a set of lat pull-downs (back). This strategy allows the muscles you just worked to rest even though you keep working. It's a great time-saving strategy if you choose to do your strength training in a gym.

- To keep your time and fuss to a minimum when lifting weights, incorporate your strength training into your daily activities. Try these simple ways to get strong all day long:

    1. Do walking lunges to your mailbox.

    2. Before you put away the groceries, use them (canned food, milk jugs, and so on) as weights. Do a set of 12 repetitions following the exercise descriptions in Chapter 11.

    3. After you do the dishes, hang around the counter just long enough to do some squats.

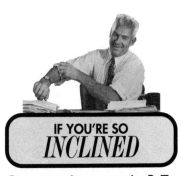

IF YOU'RE SO
INCLINED

Care to do a combo? To make the most of your moments, combine upper and lower body strength moves.

4. Carry your laundry basket with you to each room when picking up dirty clothes or putting away clean ones.

5. Do a set of step-ups before you climb the stairs.

6. Always carry your own groceries, luggage, and/or briefcase.

SHORTCUTS TO SHAPING UP YOUR DIET

It's easy to get weighed down with all of the things you should do to trim your eating. That's why I've given you the best shortcuts to shaping up your diet. Dig into the following tips, and you'll eat away at your weight:

- Cut back on fat. Fat has more than double the calories of any other nutrient (one gram of fat equals nine calories; one gram of protein or carbohydrate equals four calories). So when you shave off some fat, you slash your calorie intake.

- Cut back on sugar and refined starches (for example, white bread, white rice, and boxed pasta). If you eat too many refined sugars and/or refined starches at one meal your body will get rid of any excess blood sugar by converting and storing it as fat. Try to have no more than 8 to 15 teaspoons of added sugar a day and make sure at least half of your servings of breads/cereals/grains come from wholesome sources.

- Don't deprive yourself, but do watch your portions. Try to eat no more than two cups of food at a meal. Only take one or two bites of decadent delectables.

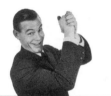

YOU'LL THANK YOURSELF LATER

You can keep yourself from overdosing on sugar by reading nutrition labels. Just take the number of grams of sugar (under carbohydrate) and divide it by four to give you the number of teaspoons per serving. Limit yourself to 8 to 15 teaspoons of added sugar daily.

- Because you won't be eating large amounts of food at a time, increase the number of times you eat during the day. Aim for eating a small meal every three to four hours (five or six meals a day) to give your body a constant supply of fuel.

- Figure out how you can drink at least 64 ounces of water every day; whether it's carrying a water bottle, keeping a pitcher in the fridge, or having a glass of water with each meal, find a way to drink your water.

- Limit your alcohol consumption. Alcohol offers no nutrients and lots of calories. Therefore, try to have no more than four drinks per week. One drink equals 12 ounces of beer, 4 ounces of wine, or 1 ounce of hard liquor.

- Fill up on fiber! Foods high in fiber (fruits, vegetables, beans, oat products, whole-grain products, and so on) tend to have fewer calories per bite than other foods and will fill you up without filling you out.

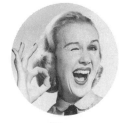

KEEPING TRACK TO GIVE YOU SOME SLACK

Keeping track of your fitness progress is important, but it shouldn't be a hassle. You can keep it from gnawing at you by having a special place for all of your logs and a specific time when you fill them out. The main thing is to make them simple. Use the ideas and sample logs in the following sections to help you track your progress with ease.

You can save yourself some time if you track your workouts as you do them (or right after). That way you won't have to back-track later.

Your Fat-Burning Log

It doesn't matter what activity you do, as long as you accumulate 30 minutes of continuous, somewhat heavy breathing at least six days a week. If you want to track your calories, you can use the table in Chapter 7.

The Fat-Burning Log

It's important to keep track of what you've done, and the easiest way to do that is to find a chart or table that will help you keep on top of the important stuff. We've put together a sample table to log the calories you've burned. Feel free to photocopy this for your own use!

The Fat-Burning Log

Week #_____

Day/Date	Aerobic Activity	Minutes	Calories

Total Minutes:_____

Total Calories:_____

Your Muscle-Building Log

It will be easy to see how much stronger you are getting when you use this log. If you use your body or elastic tubing for resistance rather than weights (dumbbells, machines, and so on), just put a *B* (body) or *T* (tubing) under *weight*.

The Muscle-Building Log

Keep a log sheet for each type of weight exercise you do, and you'll soon see your progress in black and white! Once again, this is just a sample to get you started.

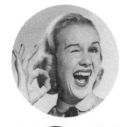

Exercise Name_____

Date _____	Set 1		Set 2	
	Weight _____		Weight _____	
	Reps _____		Reps _____	
Date _____	Set 1		Set 2	
	Weight _____		Weight _____	
	Reps _____		Reps _____	
Date _____	Set 1		Set 2	
	Weight _____		Weight _____	
	Reps _____		Reps _____	

Your Measurement Log

You'll love filling out this log every six weeks. It's a good idea to get a body composition analysis so that you can track the fat you lose as well as the inches. Make sure you reward yourself each time that you note you're melting away.

The Measurement Log

With this log sheet you should check your measurements every six weeks. More frequently can be frustrating since your body simply doesn't change that fast. With these six week increments you'll be keeping your eye on the goal and motivating yourself each time you sit down to fill in the next set of measurements!

Measurement Log

Initial Measurements

Weight _____ Body Fat % _____ Chest _____ Waist _____ Hip _____ Thigh _____

6 Week Measurements

Weight _____ Body Fat % _____ Chest _____ Waist _____ Hip _____ Thigh _____

Your Monthly Progress Report

This progress report is just a guide to help keep you on track. Use it to shape up your eating, exercise, and attitude.

The Monthly Progress Report

Not only do you need to see what you still have to work on, but when you need a little encouragement to keep going you also need to see what you've mastered. Your monthly progress report can take any form you like, be it a journal entry or a spreadsheet that you've created to keep track of how you're doing. Just make sure that you cover the important things: eating, exercise, and, most importantly, attitude. Use your monthly progress report to keep tabs on how many glasses of water you drink, what kind of foods you eat, how you feel, and which exercises you do. All of these things are crucial to get you in shape!

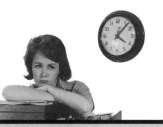

A COMPLETE WASTE OF TIME

The 3 Worst Places to Keep Your Fitness Log:

1. In the basement.

2. In the trunk of your car (under the spare tire).

3. In the trash.

Getting Time on Your Side

	The Old Way	The Lazy Way
Doing your aerobic workout	45 to 60 minutes	10 to 30 minutes
Doing your strength workout	45 to 60 minutes	5 to 30 minutes
Finding the time to exercise	30 minutes a day? No way!	5 minutes here, 5 minutes there
Logging your progress	1 hour a day	As you go!
Making up your progress reports	2 hours	2 seconds
Reaching your goals	Impossible!	You're well on your way!

The Finishing Touch

When it comes to the finishing touch, you can forget about treating yourself like a statue. There's no need for any painstaking buffing, rubbing, or polishing after you exercise. You'll shine automatically from your workouts!

You don't want to shine too much though, or you'll be likely to lose some of that sheen (a nice word for sweat) on your shoes. In this chapter, you'll find lots of tips to tidy up during and after your workouts. You'll also learn when to complete your goals and how to embark on new ones. Last, but not least, you'll get in touch with your readiness to shape up by answering a few health questions. So grab a towel and be prepared to get the rubdown on how to gear yourself to go.

A SWIPE IN TIME SAVES NINE (DROPS OF SWEAT, THAT IS)

It's not as though you're going to be sweating profusely, but wouldn't it be nice to keep the dripping to a minimum? Of course it would, and it's not that hard to do either. First, avoid

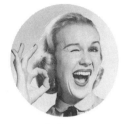

overexerting yourself. Then just follow these simple tips
to keep you cool and dry:

- The best way to stay dry if you're working out inside
  is to have a fan blowing on you. The fan will evapo-
  rate your sweat (which is a good thing). Using a fan
  makes it hard to determine just how much you do
  sweat, so be sure to drink plenty of water.

- You can keep sweat from dripping off your forehead
  and arms by wearing terry cloth bands around your
  head and wrists. These bands work great for any of
  your outdoor activities, with the exception of swimming.

- Have a towel handy for swiping sweat while exercising. Keep one underneath you when doing floor
  work, too. You can also put a towel over your head
  if you don't want to be noticed by anyone in the
  gym.

- Wearing a handkerchief or scarf that has been
  soaked in ice cold water around your neck will sop
  up your sweat and cool you off at the same time.
  Such a scarf is especially helpful when walking or
  hiking in the heat of the day.

IT JUST TAKES A PAT HERE AND THERE, BEFORE PUTTING IT IN GEAR

If you stay pretty dry during your workouts, you won't
have much grooming to do. Your biggest clean-up will
be after your 30-minute exercise sessions. The smaller
your chunks of exercise time, the quicker you can refresh

yourself after exercising. Use these wash-up tips, and you won't wash out:

- If you have the time after your 30-minute chunk of aerobic activity, you may want to take a quick shower. But if you don't have much time, wet a towel or sponge and apply it where you need it most. Don't forget the deodorant!

- You probably won't need a shower if you are exercising 10 minutes or less at a time. Keep a towel with you to wipe off any sweat. Then use moisture wipes to clean up the residue and leave you feeling refreshed.

- Always wash your hands before leaving the gym. Those machines and dumbbells come in contact with a lot of bodies and sweat. Need I say more?

- Keep an extra T-shirt with you at work. That way, if you go for a walk or decide to hit the stairwell, you only need to change your shirt or blouse (and shoes if you aren't wearing sneakers already).

A LITTLE PUSH KEEPS YOU FROM FEELING LIKE MUSH

Getting in shape *The Lazy Way* completely avoids any pain or strain, but that doesn't mean a little push now and then will do you harm. Pushing yourself with fitness goals will keep you motivated, boost your confidence, and enhance your well-being (not to mention your shape).

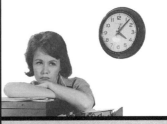

A COMPLETE WASTE OF TIME

The 3 Worst Ways to Clean Up After a Workout:

1. Take a bubble bath.

2. Spit and shine.

3. Go through a car wash with the windows rolled down.

How do you give yourself a push without it becoming a shove? The key is to set one (just one!) fitness goal for each week (see Chapter 3 for advice on setting realistic goals). Then you need to have a plan to accomplish it. For instance, if you decide you want to walk every day during your lunch hour, you'll need to determine whether you'll go before or after your lunch, make sure you bring your walking shoes to work, and maybe ask a friend or co-worker to join you. At the end of the week, examine your results. When you reach your goal, be sure to reward yourself.

As each week goes by, set more challenging goals. If you feel your workouts are getting easy or if you have more breaks in your schedule, then it's time for another push. Here are a few suggestions to keep you moving forward:

- Try a new type of workout. Check out yoga, kickboxing, water aerobics, or a new exercise video.

- Add more chunks of workout time into your day.

- Increase the intensity of your workout, but remember, it's a push, not a shove!

- Increase the length of your workout.

ONE LAST TOUCH BEFORE YOUR FIRST MOVE

You're ready to get in shape. At least you tell yourself that, but what if your body isn't ready? It's important to know if you are physically ready to start moving. It wouldn't hurt to get a check-up. But for now, please answer yes or no to the following questions:

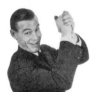

1. Has your doctor ever said you have heart trouble?

2. Has your doctor ever said your blood pressure was too high?

3. Does walking up a flight of stairs make you short of breath?

4. Do you often feel faint or have spells of dizziness?

5. Do you ever have pain, pressure, or tightness in your chest brought on by exertion?

6. Has your doctor ever told you that you have a bone, joint, muscular, or vein problem (such as arthritis, gout, bad back, or varicose veins) that is aggravated or made worse by exercising?

7. Are you over 65 and not accustomed to moderate exercise?

8. Do you smoke more than a pack of cigarettes a day?

9. Are you more than 50 pounds overweight?

10. Is there a good physical reason, not mentioned above, why you should not start an exercise program?

If you answered yes to one or more questions, consult your doctor before making your first move. If you answered no to all of the questions, then you can reasonably be sure that you are physically ready to exercise (especially *The Lazy Way*). All you have to do is read on to see how easy it is to unwhip yourself into shape.

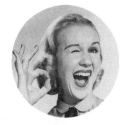

QUICK ⬛ PAINLESS

Fill out a health screen before you begin an exercise program (no matter how lazy it is). It will just take a sec, so what the heck?

Getting Time on Your Side

	The Old Way	The Lazy Way
Keeping the sweat off	All the time (Can't keep up!)	Barely ever (What sweat?)
Cleaning up after your workout	15 to 30 minutes	2 to 6 minutes
Changing your clothes	10 minutes	3 minutes
Following up on your fitness goals	Never	Every week
Taking a fitness readiness test	Day-long battery of tests (aerobic capacity, maximum rep, flexibility, and on)	2 minutes
Keeping cool while you work out	Impossible	2 seconds

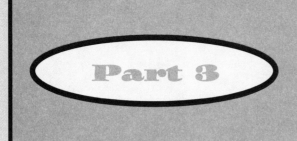

Part 3

Unwhipping You into Shape

Are You Too Lazy to Read Unwhipping You into Shape?

1 Your idea of going for a jog is running a couple of errands. ☐ yes ☐ no

2 You dream of having bulging muscles simply by guzzling a can of spinach. ☐ yes ☐ no

3 Your best stretch of the day is reaching for the remote control. ☐ yes ☐ no

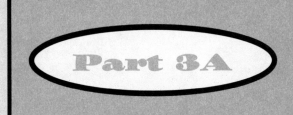

Your Aerobic Conditioning: Just a Heartbeat Away

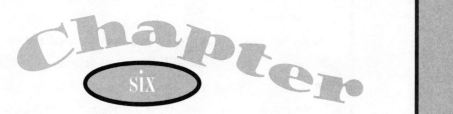

A Huff and a Puff That's Not Too Rough

Yes, you do have to huff and puff, but you don't have to blow yourself down! You just need to tune in to the bare minimum level you should work at to get results. It's somewhere above taking a bubble bath, but way below hyperventilating.

There are many reasons why you want to stay in this zone (the main one being that you need not overexert yourself). In this chapter, I'll explain the benefits of huffing and puffing along with easy ways to keep track of your heart rate. Then, I'll explain the difference between aerobic and anaerobic exercise. So take a deep breath, and let's begin.

YOU HAVE TO HUFF AND PUFF TO STRUT YOUR STUFF

If you want to reap the benefits of aerobic exercise, you will need to get a little heated, breathless, and sweaty. Getting there isn't so bad. It's kind of like jumping on the bed—you end up huffing and puffing, but you don't realize it until you stop. Don't be afraid to exert yourself a little. Exertion will change your body inside and out.

Here's why you have to huff and puff to strut your stuff:

- Working your muscles burns lots of calories and fat. The more you work muscles (the higher the percentage of intensity and duration), the more fat you burn.

- You will improve your cardiopulmonary system; your heart and lungs will strengthen, and your blood vessels will expand and stay flexible.

- Your muscles will be trained to store more glycogen (sugar). This increased storage means you will use less insulin because sugar from the blood will enter the muscle cells more quickly.

- Your aerobic exercise will help decrease stress, blood pressure, and appetite.

- Your aerobic exercise will improve endurance, balance, coordination, HDL cholesterol levels (the good cholesterol), weight loss/control, and your mood.

RESTING YOUR HEART RATE

When you are resting or relaxed, your heart beats relatively slowly and pumps relatively gently. This easy-going beat is considered your resting heart rate. There are a couple of reasons why you should acquaint yourself with your resting heart rate. First of all, you can plug this number into target heart rate zone formulas to make

QUICK ⬭ PAINLESS

The more fit your muscles are, the more fat you'll burn. The best way to get fit is by doing a combination of aerobic, strength, and flexibility exercises.

them more personalized (and dear) to your own heart. Secondly, your resting heart rate is a good indicator of your fitness level. The more fit you are (and get), the lower your resting heart rate is.

It's quite easy to determine your resting heart rate. You don't even have to get out of bed! Just lay back and relax, and find your pulse at your wrist or neck. Count the number of beats for one full minute. Do this on three different days (you can get out of bed in between), and take the average of the numbers to get your resting heart rate.

When you exercise, you usually start at your resting heart rate. This rate is a lot slower than the speed your heart beats when you're moving. That's why it's important to warm up (a heat lamp won't do the trick). The purpose of a warm-up is to gradually prepare your body for more lively exercise by slowly raising the muscular temperature and increasing blood flow to the working muscles, so be sure to begin your workout at an easy pace for three to five minutes. After you've warmed up your muscles, you can stretch them out (see Chapter 16 for some simple stretches).

If you start out slowly, you should end slowly, too! A cool-down is the gradual tapering off of activity. Its purpose is to allow the body to gradually return to normal circulation patterns. Aerobic activity increases blood flow to the lower extremities, and cooling down prevents blood from pooling in this area, away from the heart. To cool down, just do what you did for your warm-up. You'll be back at your resting heart rate before you know it.

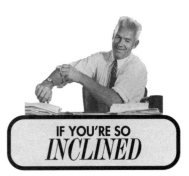

IF YOU'RE SO
INCLINED

You can get a good estimate of your average resting heart rate if you take your pulse for one minute right after you wake up. Do this at least three days during the week and then take the average.

Give yourself a few minutes to warm up before you exercise. Just do whatever activity you planned to do, but keep it at a snail's pace (okay, maybe a turtle's pace).

PICKING A ZONE OF YOUR OWN

When you work out, you need to get into a zone, a state in which your heart beats faster but not too fast. This zone is your target heart rate or target range, and it's usually measured in heartbeats per minute. You don't want to get into your zone just from trying to figure out how to measure it! That's why I'm giving you some effortless ways to help you tune in to where you need to be.

Don't Walk If You Can't Talk

The easiest way to measure whether you are in your target range is by doing the talk test. You'll know you are in your zone if you are breathing hard but can still speak easily. If it takes you a minute to spit out a sentence, you're going way too hard. The only glitch with this method is that you might get some weird looks from others if you are talking to yourself (yet another good reason to have a workout buddy!).

Behold How You Are Holding Up

Another simple way to measure whether you are on target is to tune in to your body and feel how hard you are working. For instance, if you are jogging, do you feel as though you can keep going, or do you feel like you're going backwards? Remember, you want to be just a little heated, breathless, and sweaty. Listening to your body means asking yourself how your exercise feels to you at that moment. Here is a scale to help you out:

- Very easy (like drying off after a bubble bath)
- Fairly easy
- Moderate
- Hard
- Very hard
- Very, very hard (on the verge of hyperventilating)

You want to exercise at a level that is in the middle of this scale (moderate to hard). Remember that what feels moderate today may seem very hard tomorrow, so as you exercise, pay attention to what is happening now.

Are You Worried About Zoning Out?

If you'd feel better having an actual number for your target rate, then all you have to do is count your pulse while you're exercising. This can be a little tricky to do while you're moving around, so you may have to temporarily stop to feel your pulse clearly. Instead of counting your pulse for a whole minute, just count your pulse over 10 seconds and multiply by six. Do this several times during your workout and take the lowest and highest count you get as your target range.

The table on the next page shows target training zones (60 to 85 percent) for exercising at a pace that is moderate to hard, based on age. Numbers are based on a 10-second count.

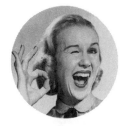

QUICK PAINLESS

If you want to be in your target zone, but you don't want to count your pulse, just ask yourself how exercising feels. If it's easy, you probably aren't in your zone. If it's medium to somewhat hard, you probably are.

If you want to determine your individual target heart rate zone using your resting heart rate, turn to Appendix C at the back of the book. Or you can just listen to your body.

Percentage of Maximum Heart Rate

Age	60%	65%	70%	75%	80%	85%
20	20	22	23	25	27	28
25	20	21	23	24	26	28
30	19	21	22	24	25	27
35	19	20	22	23	25	26
40	18	20	21	23	24	26
45	18	19	20	22	23	25
50	17	18	20	21	23	24
55	17	18	19	21	22	24
60	16	17	19	20	21	23
65	16	17	18	20	21	22
70	15	16	17	19	20	22
75	15	15	17	18	19	21

TO BE OR NOT TO BE WITHOUT OXYGEN

I'm sure if you had a choice you'd prefer to be with oxygen. After all, who would want to (or could) live without it? I guess it's more a question of how much oxygen can make a difference. Exercising at different intensities affects your oxygen uptake and what fuel your muscles use. It all depends on how much you huff and puff.

A Puffy Huff or a Huffy Puff

If you are huffing and puffing, yet you still have a lot of steam, you are probably in your target zone (60 to 85 percent of your maximum heart rate), which is considered aerobic. When you huff and puff so hard that you run out of steam (breath), you are then anaerobic. Simply put, *aerobic* means in the presence of oxygen, and *anaerobic* means without oxygen. Because you're getting in shape *The Lazy Way,* you'll be happy to know that you're staying at the aerobic level. But a few anaerobic bursts every now and then can add a lot to your fitness, even though they may take away your breath.

The benefit of doing anaerobic bursts comes not so much from the actual burst, but from the recovery period after, when your body replaces the energy it burned up. This recovery period increases your body's capacity to make and use more ATP (energy). It's definitely worth getting out of breath for!

A Short Burst Is Not a Bust

Adding some anaerobic bits in the middle of your aerobic workout can get you fitter faster, and it's easy to do.

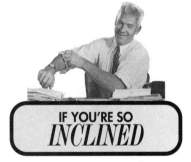

IF YOU'RE SO INCLINED

Add some anaerobic spurts to your aerobic workouts. Just push yourself for a minute or two then allow yourself to recover at a lower pace for double that time.

While exercising, go a bit faster than is comfortable (say for half a minute or a minute), and then return to your regular pace, breathing comfortably before starting another burst. This change in intensity causes your body to recover under stress, and that's what will raise your fitness level. You'll learn more about how to incorporate anaerobic intervals into your workouts in Chapter 8.

Your Duration Will Decide Your Elevation

When time is the limiting factor for your workouts, and you need to do 10-minute chunks or less, you will get better results if you increase your intensity. Don't make your workouts anaerobic, but do try to stay at the high end of your target range. The good news is that your workout will be over before you know it.

If you prefer to take it slow and easy, then you'll need to give yourself more time. Staying at the low end of your zone requires 30 minutes or more of exercise. The choice is yours: short and brisk or long and mellow.

What's Burning?!

The primary fuels for your muscles while you're exercising are sugar and fat. How much oxygen your body is taking in and delivering to your muscles will determine which fuel is used more.

Fat cannot be burned without oxygen. On the other hand, sugar can be burned without oxygen, but it does not break down completely. In order for your body to burn fat and sugar completely, your heart and lungs have to be able to supply enough oxygen to your muscles. This

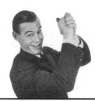

YOU'LL THANK YOURSELF LATER

If you don't have much energy, but do have the time, plan to do a longer workout at a slower pace. That way, you'll still get your exercise in without getting too red in the face!

is achieved when you work out aerobically in your target range (65 to 80 percent of your maximum heart rate).

Your anaerobic bursts will only burn sugar for those moments, but as you slow down your pace, you'll burn lots of fat to replace the energy you used up. But don't get caught up in what you burn, just make sure you move your muscles so that you burn something!

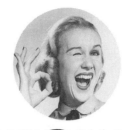

QUICK ⊂▪▪▶ PAINLESS

If you want to light your fat furnace, then you need to keep the oxygen flowing. That means you have to keep on blowing without blowing yourself out!

Getting Time on Your Side

	The Old Way	The Lazy Way
Warming up	10 minutes	3 to 5 minutes
Cooling down	10 minutes	3 to 5 minutes
Checking your resting heart rate	1 minute	15 seconds
Checking your target heart rate	1 minute	10 seconds
Finding your target zone	5 minutes	30 seconds
Staying anaerobic	A whole workout	1 to 2 minutes at a time

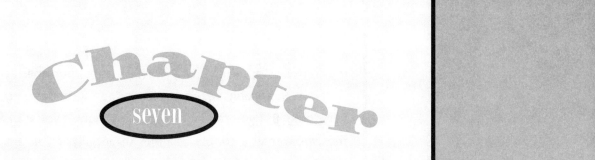

Fat-Burning Movin' That Feels Like Groovin'

Fat-burning moving is like riding a merry-go-round. You glide in a constant rhythm as your surroundings fade into a blur. Yet you know you'll never go so fast that you'll get dizzy. Of course, you have to move your large muscle groups, not just sit on them, to bring about this effect. But you get the idea.

Aerobic exercise consists of moving the large muscle groups of the body in a continuous and rhythmic manner. Remember, this exercise is the ticket to increasing your aerobic capacity and becoming a better fat burner. So it's important that this fat-burning movin' feels like groovin' all year long. In this chapter, you'll discover a variety of aerobic activities at all different levels. Plus, you'll find out how you can keep moving no matter what the season.

PUT YOUR REAR INTO GEAR

To get aerobic, you not only have to move your large muscle groups (that's your rear, dear), you also have to keep them

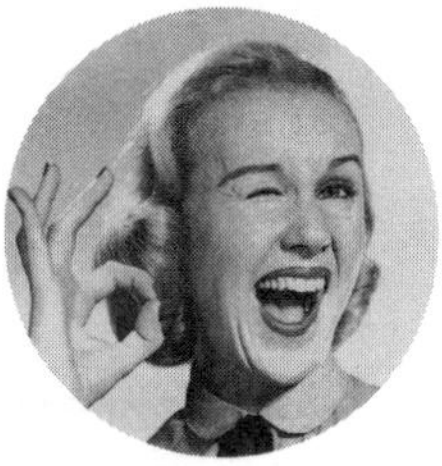

QUICK 'n' PAINLESS

Want to go steady? Fat-burning moving uses the large muscle groups in a steady and continuous manner.

moving nonstop. That's why window shopping doesn't count as an aerobic activity—there's too much stopping and going. But you can make shopping count if you walk the whole mall a couple of times (especially if you are carrying your purchases).

When you can't keep your aerobic exercise constant, you can still get the aerobic benefit if you do a lot of it. This rule holds true for many sports activities, such as volleyball, basketball, and racquet sports. You can either play them longer or make them harder (for example, two-man team volleyball, three-on-three basketball, or singles tennis, racquetball, squash, or badminton).

There are lots of moves you can choose to put your rear into gear. All you need to do is decide where you want to go and how much you want to rev it up. The following activities are organized according to different intensity levels. Pick the ones that suit you best.

If You Want to Coast

Taking it easy is probably not going to get you into your target zone, but sometimes taking it easy is what you need to do. This is especially true if you are injured or feeling under the weather. (If you are sick, you should stay in bed!) Also, when you are just beginning an exercise program, you should always start out slowly and build up gradually.

Try these moves if you want to coast:

- Walking (easy)
- Walking in the shallow end of a pool
- Marching in place

- Stationary cycling (easy)
- Doing an exercise video (beginning level)
- Swimming (easy)
- Tai chi
- Jumping on a minitrampoline
- Un-workouts (see Chapter 9)

Grooving Without Grinding

Grooving without grinding is like humming down the highway while going the speed limit. This exercise is just moderate to somewhat hard on your engine, so you can keep the motion steady and continuous. When you groove without the grind, you have no problem staying in your target zone. The only thing you need for the long haul is to make sure you have a variety of moves (you need to have a change of scenery to avoid highway hypnosis).

Choose from these activities to groove into your target zone:

- Stationary cycling
- Running on a treadmill
- Using a stair stepper
- Rowing on a rowing machine
- Using an exercise rider
- Swimming
- Doing water aerobics
- Brisk walking
- Hiking

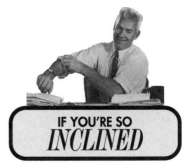

IF YOU'RE SO
INCLINED

If you're feeling under the weather, take it easy on yourself and do your exercise in slow motion. If you're really feeling sick, don't even bother moving.

- Jogging/running
- Aerobic dancing
- Ice and roller skating

You Might Need a Push

There will be times when you'll want to push yourself (believe it or not). Maybe you had a great night's sleep or too much coffee. Whatever the reason, the activities at this level are very challenging and not ones for conversation (you'll be lucky if you can breathe).

Because these activities are intense, they should be short-lived with lots of recovery time in between. You can sustain them longer if you take the intensity down a few notches. Just remember, if you get to the point when you're gasping for breath, it's time to put it in neutral and recover.

These activities will give you a push:

- Running sprints
- Running stairs
- Cross-country skiing
- Moving up mountains (hiking, biking)
- Jumping rope
- Outdoor rowing (fast pace)

Checking the Fuel Gauge

Those of you who like to watch the fuel gauge will probably enjoy seeing how much fuel you burn when you go the distance. Of course, the faster and longer you go, the more calories you burn. The following table shows the

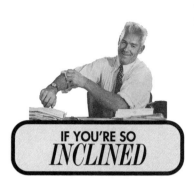

Calories Expended During 30-Minute Workouts

Activity	120 pounds	140 pounds	160 pounds	180 pounds	200 pounds
Basketball	205	239	273	307	341
Bicycling	105	120	138	155	173
Canoeing	108	126	144	162	180
Dancing, aerobic	252	294	336	378	420
Dancing, ballroom	72	84	96	108	120
Fencing	144	168	192	216	240
Hiking	160	185	211	237	264
Jogging (10-minute mile)	274	319	365	410	456
Jumping rope	235	273	313	352	397
Kayaking	90	105	120	135	150
Martial arts	216	252	288	324	360
Ping-Pong	101	121	139	156	174
Rowing	210	245	279	314	349
Running (8-minute mile)	342	399	456	513	570
Skating, ice	162	189	216	243	270
Skating, roller	198	231	264	297	330
Skiing, cross-country	360	420	480	540	600
Swimming	218	255	294	331	368
Tennis, singles	162	189	216	243	270
Volleyball	144	168	192	216	240
Walking (4 miles per hour)	146	171	195	220	244

calories expended over 30 minutes for various activities
(at a grooving without grinding pace) for people of different weights.

IT'S THE TIME OF THE SEASON FOR MOVING

Just because the season changes doesn't mean you have
to give up your exercise. Use the change of season as an
opportunity to get your feet wet (not frozen) and acclimate yourself to whatever activities the season may
offer. Whether it's winter, spring, summer, or fall, try a
new activity, no matter how small.

Coming Out of Hibernation

When winter rolls around, so does the snow (unless you
live in a no snow zone), and that means it's the time for
scraping windows, throwing snowballs, and making
snow angels. There are many exciting activities you can
do in the snow as long as you have the equipment and
time to go.

One of the precautions you need to take during this
time of year is to protect yourself from the cold (especially the wind chill). Dress in layers when you work out
and make sure you keep your hands, feet, ears, and face
warm! Keep some lip balm handy for your lips, too. If the
weather and temperatures are too miserable, you might
want to have some indoor alternatives for your exercise.

These activities fit the bill for working out in a chill:

- Skiing (downhill or cross-country)
- Snow boarding

- Snowshoeing
- Ice skating
- Shoveling snow
- Mall walking (indoor)
- Doing exercise videos (indoor)

Keeping Your Spring from Getting Sprung

Spring is a wonderful season when flowers bud and bloom. But it's also that time of year when you're supposed to clean up every room. (Don't worry! You can clean your house *The Lazy Way!*) The early mornings can be quite chilly, so you might want to wait until the middle of the day to work out. If you tend to get bad allergy attacks, avoid exercising outside on windy days. Don't let a little rain stop you though, just be sure to take a nice hot shower when you finish your exercise.

Spring into action with these fun activities (minus the mandatory clean-ups):

- Hiking
- Mountain biking
- Inline skating
- Tennis
- Gardening
- Pruning
- Spring cleaning

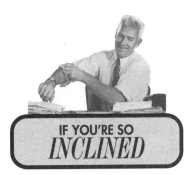

IF YOU'RE SO
INCLINED

Plan to spring clean your house for one (or many) of your workouts. Be sure to put on some lively music to boost your cleaning power.

Hot! Hot! Hot! Not! Not! Not!

There's nothing better than spending your summer near water. Not only does it keep you cool, but it also offers a playground for having fun and being active. Now's the time to reward yourself with a new swimsuit for continuing your exercise since New Year's.

Summer can be a scorcher, so make sure you protect yourself with sunscreen, sunglasses, and a hat. Drink plenty of water, too! The more you sweat, the more you need to rehydrate yourself.

Check out these hot activities for summer:

- Swimming
- Water aerobics
- Water skiing
- Boogie boarding/body surfing
- Kayaking
- Canoeing
- Rock climbing
- Volleyball

Free-Falling

Fall brings lots of changes: shorter days, brilliant foliage, and often some drizzle. There's no other time of year when you can feel the leaves crunch under your steps or get a great workout raking them up. If the darker days get you blue, try some new indoor group activities to raise your spirits (and your heart rate). 'Tis also the season for holiday treats. So make sure you burn extra calories to cover the extras that may enter your lips.

Here's how to give it your all this fall:

- Brisk walks
- Bike trips (for autumn foliage)

A COMPLETE WASTE OF TIME

The 3 Worst Things to Do When Exercising in the Sun:

1. Forget to apply sunscreen.

2. Forget to drink water.

3. Forget to wear clothes.

- Racquetball
- Basketball
- Dance classes (swing, ballroom, line, and so on)
- Martial arts
- Fencing
- Raking leaves
- Raking leaves
- Raking leaves

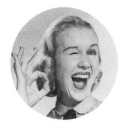

Getting Time on Your Side

	The Old Way	The Lazy Way
Choosing your aerobic activity	5 minutes (and you still end up doing the same old thing)	A second
Planning your winter exercise	A whole season	A few weeks
Planning your spring exercise	A whole season	A few weeks
Planning your summer exercise	A whole season	A few weeks
Planning your fall exercise	A whole season	A few weeks
Figuring your calories burned	30 minutes (not counting the drive to the library)	2 to 5 minutes

Mix It Up to Slim Down

The deciding moment came when you waved for a taxi and noticed your arm kept on waving. Determined to get rid of the jiggle, you subject yourself to a gazillion arm exercises. Day and night you work those arms hoping to zap the fat, but you find the only thing that keeps them from jiggling is that they're too sore to even move!

If it's not your arms, it's your thighs or hips or stomach. Don't feel bad about this—after all, it's human nature to zero in on your "erodenous" zones. The problem is you can't just work on one specific spot and expect it to melt away. Your body fat has a mind of its own (along with some input from previous generations), and it decides when and where it will disappear.

But don't give up hope! You can speed up the slimming down process with cross-training and interval training and by making the most of your chunks of exercise time. Mix these ingredients into your routine, and you'll shape up in no time.

CROSS-TRAINING: A FAR CRY FROM BOOT CAMP

Cross-training sounds heavy-duty, but it makes the whole process of exercising easier on you. All cross-training means is doing a variety of different exercises as your fitness routine. Cross-training will help you combine moderate, rhythmic movements; intense, rapid movements; soft, relaxing movements; and static, balancing movements.

Here's why you'll want to enlist in some cross-training:

- When you cross-train, you work many different sets of muscles. The more muscles you use, the more fat you burn.

- Cross-training decreases the chances of injury because you're not using the same muscle groups all the time.

- You'll be less bored if you have a variety of exercises to choose from. You can even alternate indoor and outdoor activities.

- Cross-training can broaden your sense of adventure. Whether you train for an event or choose a recreational sport (such as skiing, rock climbing, or mountain biking) to challenge you, learning something new keeps your exercise fun and motivating.

- Remember, doing only one kind of exercise increases some aspects of body fitness, but decreases others. For example, doing only aerobics can lessen the ability of muscles to perform strength tasks; and doing

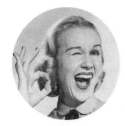

QUICK ⬤ PAINLESS

Here's a deduction about spot reduction: Don't waste your time and effort focusing on one problem area because it doesn't work. Get rid of that notion, along with your cellulite-removal potion.

only strength exercises decreases the body's endurance. That's why aerobic, strength, and flexibility exercises all need to be part of your routine.

Mix it up, and you'll have no problem slimming down. It can be as simple as walking one day, swimming for the next workout, and doing some strength exercises as you clean the house later in the week.

YOU CAN BURST WITH ENERGY IF YOU TAKE A BREAK

If you are gung-ho to rev up your fat burning, then you need to add a few bursts of speed. (Don't forget the pit stops!) These bursts are part of *interval training*. I'll give you some routines to help get you started, but first let's look at some guidelines for interval training:

1. Do not begin interval training until you have established an aerobic base. You need to be able to exercise comfortably for at least 30 minutes.

2. Always be completely warmed up before starting your intervals. It's best to be exercising aerobically for at least 10 to 15 minutes before increasing your intensity.

3. Go at your own level. When you are out of air, it's time to stop and catch your breath.

4. The number of times you repeat an interval is up to you. It can be as little as three or as many as eight. If you notice you can't keep up the pace, then you've probably done enough.

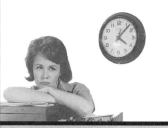

A COMPLETE WASTE OF TIME

The 3 Worst Ways to Cross-Train:

1. Do only strength workouts one week, and then do only aerobic workouts the next week.

2. Compete in an Ironman Triathlon.

3. Wear a different type of sneaker on each foot.

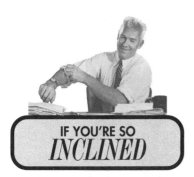

5. The more intense the interval, the longer your recovery time should be. Do not start another interval until you are completely recovered.

Follow the routines in the following sections, and you'll get fitter, faster.

Find a Hill

Hills are a sure bet for raising your heart rate. If you don't live in a mountainous area, you can always go to the nearest (safe) overpass.

1. Pick a spot on the hill about 50 yards up from your starting point. The fitter you are, the longer the distance can be.

2. Run up the hill, pacing yourself so that you can make it to your end point.

3. Turn around and walk back down. Keep walking until your heart rate is back to normal. Repeat the interval.

Pick a Lightpost or Telephone Pole

When you are on a walk or run, you can use lightposts or telephone poles as markers to jog or sprint between.

1. If you are walking, increase your pace to a very brisk walk or jog. If you are running, make it a sprint. Do this for the distance between two poles, concentrating on your form as you go.

2. Take the distance between the next three or four poles to recover. Walk or jog slowly, bringing your heart rate back down. Repeat the interval.

Spin Your Wheels

You can do intervals on your bike, too. They just need to be longer than the distance between two telephone poles. If you are on a stationary bike, you can program it to increase the resistance for your intervals.

1. It's easier to measure your intervals by time instead of distance when on the bike. Do a hard sprint (90 to 95 percent of your maximum heart rate) for 30 seconds to 1 minute.

2. Recover by spinning slowly for three minutes. Then repeat the sprint.

Climb the Stairs

Whether you take stairs one or two at a time, climbing them will take your heart rate to new heights. Make sure you bring it down to ground level before taking off again.

1. Find a stairwell in a building with lots of stories. You can also use a single flight of stairs (12 to 15), but you will have to run up and down them as part of the interval.

2. Run up three flights or to the point where you are out of breath.

3. Turn around and slowly walk back down the stairs. Do not repeat the interval until your breathing is normal!

4. You can vary this interval routine by taking the stairs two at a time or turning to the right 45 degrees for a flight and then to the left 45 degrees for the next set of stairs.

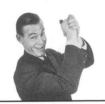

YOU'LL THANK YOURSELF LATER

The next time you're on the stationary bike, warm up the seat a little more by increasing the resistance and doing some short intervals. You'll keep burning calories long after you're through spinning.

Dive into the Pool

Intervals aren't just for dry land. You can sprint some laps in the pool, too. The great thing about pool workouts is that your legs won't take a pounding.

1. Swim one lap at a medium pace (80 to 85 percent of your maximum heart rate).

2. Swim the next lap at a fast pace (90 to 95 percent).

3. Recover by swimming a lap at an easy pace (60 to 65 percent).

4. Take a 30-second break, then repeat the interval set (medium, fast, slow).

Now you have a few routines to help you burst with energy. Just remember to take a break between intervals and an even longer one after you're done. Make sure a few days go by before you rev it up again.

MAKE THE MOST OF YOUR CHUNKS

If your workout time is limited, you'll have to push your limit a little. The key is to choose challenging activities you can do on the spot. There's always a brisk walk, but that can get dull after a while. These moves will make the most of your exercise chunks (and cheeks!):

- Get out your jump rope. Be sure to alternate your moves (such as double skip, single skip, switching legs, and so on).

- Visit your nearest stairwell and start climbing. You can take the steps one or two at a time. Just make sure you don't overstep your target heart rate range.

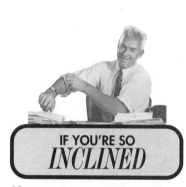

IF YOU'RE SO INCLINED

If you want to get in a good interval workout when you're traveling, just find the stairwell in your hotel. Run up as many flights as you can (or want) and walk back down to recover (or you could always take the elevator).

- Skip around the block. You'll burn a few more calories if you whistle too!

- Move around the gym. Pick three or four different cardio machines and just spend a few minutes on each one.

- Add some strength to your aerobic moves. For instance, do a few minutes on the stationary bike, and then do a set of lunges. Or put on some wrist weights when you go for a walk to give your arms a pump.

- Do some jumping jacks. You can make them interesting by changing arm movements and facing different directions.

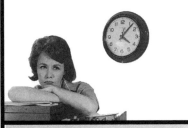

A COMPLETE WASTE OF TIME

The 3 Worst Ways to Slim Down After Dinner:

1. Have seconds.
2. Sit on the couch and watch television.
3. Purge the food.

Getting Time on Your Side

	The Old Way	**The Lazy Way**
Adding some cross-training	Adds extra days	Doesn't change a thing
Combining aerobics and strength workouts	1 to 2 hours	10 to 30 minutes
Stimulating your metabolism	Hours	Minutes
Doing a hard workout	30 to 40 minutes	10-minute chunks
Resting between intervals	5 to 10 minutes	2 to 4 minutes
Burning extra calories	Days	Minutes

The Un-Workout

Of course it's never a lack of will that keeps you from working out. (Heaven forbid I even suggested that!) Rather, it's usually a lack of time. You always have the best intentions, yet sometimes the only exercise you can fit in is going to the bathroom. On days when even a 10-minute exercise chunk is out of the question, your best bet is doing the un-workout.

The un-workout involves making a conscious decision to keep moving so that you can unconsciously burn more calories with your daily activities (such as being all you can be, sitting down). The un-workout can even shape you up during your downtime or when you are traveling. Small moves can make a big difference.

SEVEN WAYS TO UNCONSCIOUSLY BURN MORE CALORIES IN YOUR DAY

In our modern society we have no time to waste, nor unnecessary energy to expend, so we have learned to do things with the least possible effort. As everything gets faster, we become slower.

It doesn't have to be this way. All you need to do is find a way to be more active while doing your daily activities. The following seven ideas will help keep you moving:

■ Wean yourself from technology. Modern conveniences are not efficient at making you burn more calories. Your body is better off when you do things the old-fashioned way. Here are a dozen ways to wean yourself from technology:

1. Mix and/or beat your batter with a wooden spoon.

2. Blow off the blower and rake your leaves.

3. Sharpen your knives by hand (and a sharpening stone, of course).

4. Shine your own shoes.

5. Always take the stairs over the escalator or elevator.

6. Put away your bread machine and knead the dough yourself.

7. Slice and dice with a knife instead of a Cuisinart.

8. Mow your lawn with an old-fashioned push mower.

9. Crank on a manual can opener.

10. Use a separate shampoo and conditioner instead of a combo (scrub extra long).

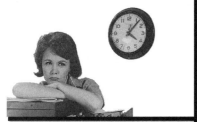

A COMPLETE WASTE OF TIME

The 3 Worst Reasons to Not Work Out:

1. Not enough time.

2. Just don't have the time.

3. Can't find the time.

If you have the time to breathe, you have the time to work out!

11. Make your popcorn over the stove.

12. Go to the library instead of surfing the Internet.

- Don't be afraid to make extra trips. Forget about piling everything at the bottom of the stairs for a solitary ascent. You don't have to wait for more than one reason to go down to the basement either. When you clear the table, do it one place setting at a time; the more trips you make, the more dinner you wear off!

- Take active commercial breaks. When watching TV, make sure you move around during the commercials. You can stretch, do a set of jumping jacks, or finish some chores. If you prefer to stay seated, choose from some of the exercises later in this chapter (for example, ABC's, pedal pushers, thigh flaps, and so on).

- Park farther away. Instead of wasting time circling around the parking lot looking for the closest space, choose to park at least the length of one football field away. Whenever you have errands that are close to home, leave your car parked in the garage and walk or bike the short distance.

- Tackle uncompleted tasks. Need something done around the house or office? Instead of looking for volunteers, roll up your sleeves and do it yourself. Whether it's changing a light bulb, adding more toner or chopping some firewood, embrace any task because it all adds up. Take a look at how many calories some common household chores use up in just 15 minutes.

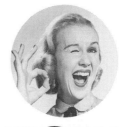

QUICK 🔘 *PAINLESS*

Ditch the remote control! If you want to change the channel, get up and push the button on the television. This change will either increase your trips from the couch to the TV or decrease your channel surfing.

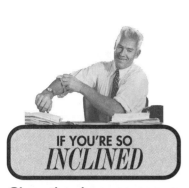

Get out in the yard. There are so many ways you can burn calories in your own back (or front) yard. You can pull weeds, trim trees, plant plants, or dig dirt if you want, or you could wipe off the chaise lounge before your afternoon snooze.

Play active games. Instead of sitting down for a game of bridge or Monopoly, choose active games such as horseshoes, croquet, Frisbee, or hopscotch.

Drive right by the drive-throughs. Nowadays there are drive-throughs for almost everything: eating,

Making Those Chores Count!

Chore	Approximate Expended Calories in 15 Minutes (Based on a 140-Pound Person)
Making beds	30
Washing dishes	30
Ironing	30
Putting groceries away	40
Vacuuming	50
Washing car	50
Weeding	50
Chopping firewood (the old-fashioned way)	90
Shoveling snow	100

banking, dry cleaning, and even getting married. Do yourself a favor and park (far away). You'll probably save time by going in, because everyone else is in the drive-through, saving their calories.

BE ALL THAT YOU CAN BE SITTING DOWN

It seems the more technology advances, the more time we spend in (and on) our seats. This constant sitting can be detrimental to your shape, especially the lower half, but not if you incorporate a few easy moves and simple guidelines for your sitting down time.

These Moves Work Best When You Recline

There are a couple of exercises you wouldn't dare try when standing. You'd get a lot more out of them if you just sat back and relaxed. The next time you're on the couch or a park bench, give these two moves a try:

- Do your ABCs. Scoot your fanny forward so that it rests at the edge of your seat. Lean back, keeping your abdominals pulled in, and extend your legs in front of you. Using both legs, begin tracing the alphabet. You can do it with capital or small-cased letters in print or in cursive, or do one set of each.

- Be a pedal pusher. Scoot your fanny forward so that it rests at the edge of your seat. Lean back, keeping your abdominals pulled in, and extend your legs in front of you. Start pedaling them as if you were riding a bicycle. Don't forget to breathe and keep your abdominals pulled in tightly. Pedal for 20 to 30 cycles.

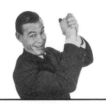

YOU'LL THANK YOURSELF LATER

Give yourself five a day—five weeds, that is. Pull five weeds from your yard every day. Before you know it, your yard will look great, and you didn't even have to break a sweat.

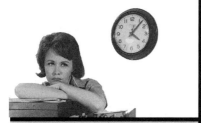

Get an Itch to Fidget

Fidgeting while you sit is an effortless way to help you burn more calories, enhance your circulation, and lighten the stress load on your back. It's a great thing to do when you're stuck in traffic, in a long meeting, or on the couch. So get an itch to fidget! These classic fidgeting moves will help you get started:

- **Thigh Flaps:** Keeping your feet flat on the floor and your abdominals pulled in, move your thighs toward the center of your body and then move them outward. Repeat continuously.

- **Jitter Bugs:** Come up on the balls of your feet and move your legs as if you are shivering or trembling. Place your palms on your thighs and start rolling your shoulders back as you continue to move your legs.

- **Toe Taps:** Keeping your left foot flat on the floor and your abdominals pulled in, flex your right foot so that it rests on your right heel then bring it down tapping your foot on the floor. Now do your left foot. Keep repeating this sequence.

- **Roly-Polys:** Move from side to side on your chair, raising your hip up toward the ceiling. Repeat continuously.

Decrees of the Throne

When you have to sit for long periods of time, you'll feel better if you follow these simple rules:

1. Never sit more than 30 or 40 minutes without getting up and moving around. Sometimes following

this guideline is a little impossible (like when you're in the center of the row at the movies). If you can't get up, be sure to do a lot of fidgeting.

2. Never settle into one position. Vary your seated positions every 15 minutes or so to lessen the stress on your back and maintain your posture. Turn to Chapter 14 for exercises and tips to prevent poor posture while sitting.

DOWNTIME MANEUVERS

No matter how busy the day is there are always a few lulls when you can catch your breath. These downtimes usually happen while you are waiting for something—a fax, a printout, the water to boil, or someone who has put you on hold. It's the perfect time to take advantage of the un-workout. Try the maneuvers described in the following sections to make the most of your downtimes.

The Un-Jumping Jack

Un-jumping jacks are great for downtime in the copy room, at the fax machine, or during commercials.

1. Stand with your feet shoulder-width apart and the palms of your hands touching your thighs.

2. Raise your arms up over your head, bringing your palms together.

3. Bring your arms back down to your thighs.

4. Repeat several times.

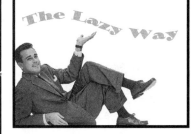

The Single Swinger

You can do the single swinger at your kitchen counter while the microwave nukes your food or even at the bathroom sink when you brush your teeth.

1. Stand next to a table or counter.

2. Turn to the right so your left hand is on the surface for support.

3. Keep your hips even and your tummy tucked and begin swinging your right leg (keep it straight) first in front and then in back like a pendulum. Your supporting left leg should be slightly bent at the knee.

4. After 10 swings, turn and switch over to the other leg.

The Comfy Cat Stretch

You'll feel a good stretch through your arm sockets with this move. The comfy cat stretch is a purrfect one for downtime while your computer prints or the credit card company has you hanging on hold.

1. Stand behind a sturdy chair or desk.

2. Place both hands on the surface, shoulder-width apart.

3. Step back, bending at the waist, and drop your head forward, keeping your chin close to your chest.

4. Push your rear back as if someone were pulling your tail.

Congratulations! You finally got the copy machine all to yourself! Go ahead and lean on it to do some downtime exercises while you make copies.

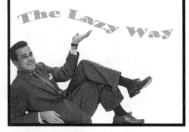

The Lazy Way

The Stationary Jogger

Use this one for lulls behind shopping carts or in front of ATM machines:

1. Stand up straight as if you were being pulled up by a string.

2. Bend the right knee, rolling the weight of your leg to the ball of your foot and bringing your right heel up.

3. Now roll back down on your heel, bending your left knee at the same time.

4. Alternate legs, rolling back in forth from toe to heel.

5. To burn a couple extra calories, swing the opposite arm when the opposite leg bends.

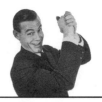

YOU'LL THANK YOURSELF LATER

The next time someone puts you on hold, put them on the speaker phone. That way, you can free up your hands (and straighten your neck) to do some feel-good stretches.

DON'T WORRY ABOUT UNRAVELING WHEN YOU'RE TRAVELING

We often bid bon voyage to our workouts whenever we travel. After all, we leave the equipment and the familiar fitness routine behind. But your shape doesn't have to unravel when you travel. You can depend on your un-workouts to keep you intact. Use these un-workout tips to nudge your hips when taking trips:

- If you're waiting for a flight at the airport, take advantage of the sprawling corridors. Instead of letting the moving sidewalks and escalators propel you forward, take the stairs and walk as much as you can. Carrying your luggage is an extra bonus.

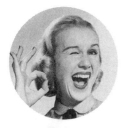

- Speaking of luggage, when you need to pick yours up from the baggage claim, head for the far end of the carousel. That way, you won't have to fight the crowds (although you could burn a few calories doing this), and you'll carry your luggage a little longer.

- When you have to sit a lot during travel, remember to change your positions frequently and never sit more than half an hour without getting up.

- Drink plenty of water especially when traveling by plane (it's very dehydrating). That way you'll stay hydrated and increase your chances for getting an un-workout by going to the bathroom (especially when traveling by plane).

- You can always depend on your own body to give you a workout. You take your legs with you wherever you go, so be sure to use them as much as you can (remember to pack your sneakers). If you want to get in some strength training, just turn to the next chapter to find several simple ways to use your body as resistance.

Getting Time on Your Side

	The Old Way	The Lazy Way
Recirculating your blood (after sitting all day)	15 minutes	1 minute
Getting luggage to your room	Arrives 5 minutes after you	Arrives instantly (with you)
Weeding your yard	2 whole days	5 minutes at a time
Completing necessary tasks	Never get done	2 minutes
Putting the shopping cart away	1 minute	30 seconds
Working out while traveling	60 minutes	10 to 30 minutes

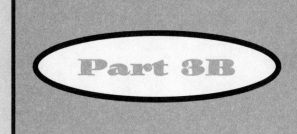
Your Muscle Strengthening: Building Up Without Breaking Down

Prod Your Bod

One piece of equipment is a must-have when shaping up *The Lazy Way.* This incredible machine is cheap, convenient, and long-lasting—in fact, it has a lifetime guarantee! You can take it with you wherever you go, and it has everything you need for your aerobic, strength, and flexibility workouts. The best thing about this extraordinary piece of equipment is that you already own it—it's your body!

You can use your body for any exercise (I guess you kind of have to), but it's especially useful as a resistance tool for strength training. Using your body for resistance forces it to stabilize itself (rather than a machine), thereby improving your balance and coordination. Using your body for resistance also allows you to work several muscle groups at once, shortening your workout time. This chapter is packed with simple and effective exercises to prod your whole bod. I'll even show you how to get strong while staying still or taking a stroll.

A FEW POINTERS BEFORE FLEXING YOUR MUSCLES

Whether you use weights, machines, elastic tubing, or your body for resistance while strength training, there are some guidelines you should follow to get the maximum benefit from your training. First, you don't have to spend hours pumping up every single muscle in your body. Here are some other guidelines to keep in mind as you begin your muscle building:

- You need to do strength training only two to three times per week.

- You don't need to do lots of sets or repetitions. Stick to 1 or 2 sets of 12 to 15 repetitions.

- Your last three repetitions should be hard to do. When they get easy, it's time to increase the weight (or add more repetitions if you are using your body as resistance).

- Rest your muscles at least 48 hours after strength exercises.

- Use proper breathing. Exhale during the hard part of the exercise and inhale during the easy part.

- Pay attention to your form. Are you aligned properly? Are your abdominals pulled in? Are you moving in a slow, controlled manner? When you use proper form, you avoid injury and ensure that you are exercising the targeted muscle.

- Stop immediately if you experience any pain. Exercise should not be painful; if it is, you're doing something wrong, probably overdoing it.

- Always keep your abdominal muscles pulled in and stabilize your body with all exercises.

- Never strength train or stretch your muscles without warming up first. (For example, do 5 to 10 minutes of easy walking before your aerobic workout.)

PROD YOUR UPPER BOD

It doesn't take many exercises to strengthen your upper torso when you use your body for resistance because you never work just one muscle at a time. The following exercises are some of the most effective strengthening moves for your upper body.

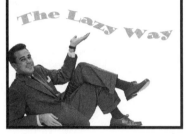

Congratulations! You've paid attention to your form, and learned to do proper breathing while you exercise! Treat yourself to a massage!

The Lazy Way

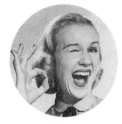
Lounging Lizard Lifts

This exercise is for your chest, shoulders, and triceps. If you have never done a lounging lizard lift (push-up) before, you may want to start out by standing up and pushing against a wall. Those of you who really want to challenge yourselves can balance your weight on your hands and feet instead of doing them on your knees.

1. Kneel on all fours on a padded floor, with your hands about shoulder-width apart and positioned slightly forward of your shoulders and your feet facing back with toes touching the floor.

2. Press your hips down to keep your torso in a straight line and keep your abdominals pulled in.

3. Slowly bend your elbows and lower your body as a unit; your chest and chin move down to nearly touch the floor. Then push back up. Don't lock your elbows.

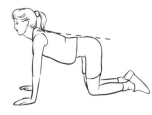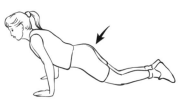

Lounging lizard lifts.

Upside-Down Lounging Lizard Lifts

Doing lounging lizard lifts upside down (on your back) will work the muscles of your back as well as your arms and shoulders. Make sure you find a table that can hold your weight.

1. Lie on your back under a heavy and sturdy table.

2. Grasp an edge of the table firmly and raise your body, using your arms. Go as far up as possible, and then sink evenly back down again.

3. Make sure your arms come back down all the way between repetitions.

4. For the beginner level of this exercise, keep your legs bent at the knees. For the advanced level, keep your legs straight and use a wide grip (your hands gripping opposite edges of the table, if possible).

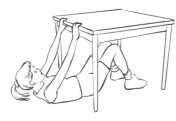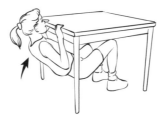

Upside-down lounging lizard lifts.

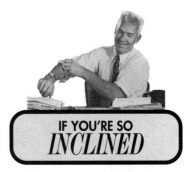

IF YOU'RE SO
INCLINED

If you want to get more out of your push-ups, do them on your hands and feet instead of on your hands and knees. That's the way to be all that you can be (without being in the army).

Dip-Downs

This exercise is great for your whole upper body. It works your chest, shoulder, triceps, and back. You will need two sturdy chairs for dip-downs.

1. Position yourself between two sturdy, stable chairs that are about two feet apart. Your knees should be bent, and your feet should be flat on the floor in front of you.

2. Slowly lower yourself by bending your arms (with your elbows moving out to the sides) until you feel a gentle stretch on your chest muscles. As you lower yourself, keep the tops of your shoulders down; don't let them rise toward your ears. Don't lock your elbows.

3. Slowly extend your arms and push yourself back up to the starting position.

4. When this exercise gets easy, you can challenge yourself by extending your legs in front of you.

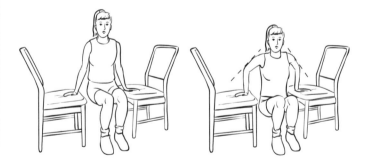

Dip-downs.

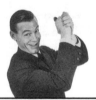

YOU'LL THANK YOURSELF LATER

Make sure you use sturdy and stable tables and chairs when doing pull-ups and dips. The last thing you need is to get out of breath because you have a piece of furniture on top of you.

PROD YOUR LOWER BOD

You're not going to work just one muscle with any of the exercises for your lower bod either. You can be assured that if you work your thighs, you'll be working your buttocks, too. Just try the following exercises, and you'll see what I mean.

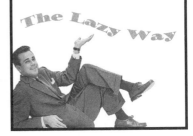

Congratulations! You've prodded your upper bod! Grab a tall glass of water and enjoy a nice break outside—it's time to smell the roses!

Kneel-Downs

Kneel-downs are great for strengthening your thighs and buttocks. They also do wonders for your balance. Once you get the hang of this exercise, you can challenge your-self by moving forward, alternating your legs with each kneel-down.

1. Stand with your feet slightly apart, toes forward, knees relaxed, and arms down at your sides.

2. Move one foot forward with your back leg balancing on the ball of the back foot. Your back heel should be off the floor, and your back knee should be slightly bent. This is your starting position.

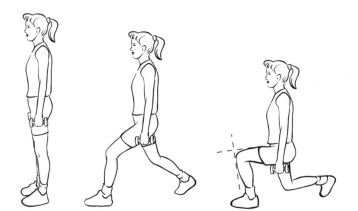

Kneel-downs.

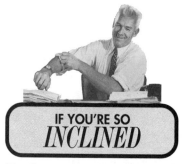

3. Start lowering your body to the floor by bending your front knee. Come down as if you were balancing a jug of water on your head, keeping your shoulders over your hips and your front knee aligned with your front foot. Keep your arms at your sides.

4. Return to the starting position and repeat the exercise for the desired number of repetitions.

5. Change legs and repeat this exercise. (You can also do this exercise with weights.)

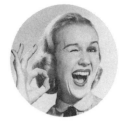

QUICK ⬤ PAINLESS

Think right—angles that is. Always try to keep your leg bent at a right angle (90 degrees) when bending your knees.

Step-Ups

You can do this exercise whenever you come across a step or low bench. You want the step or bench to be 12 to 18 inches high and stable enough to hold your body weight. If you're using a step, make sure the flat part is wide enough to place your entire foot on.

1. Lift your right foot on the step; then lift your left foot onto the step also.

2. Come down with your right foot and then your left.

3. Repeat this sequence, starting with your right foot first, for the desired amount of time.

4. Then start the exercise again with your left foot.

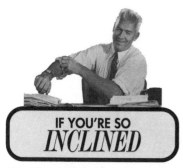

IF YOU'RE SO
INCLINED

Don't walk! But do step up! The next time you're waiting for the walk sign to flash, go ahead and step off the curb, but get right back on. Keep stepping off and on until you can step off and go!

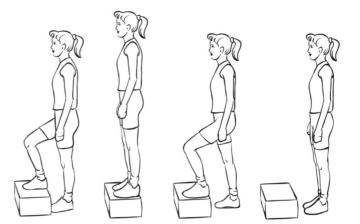

Step-ups.

Sit-Downs

Sit-downs strengthen your thighs and buttocks. They're the perfect exercise to do after you wash the dishes or brush your teeth.

1. Stand erect in front of a counter with your feet about shoulder-width apart, your toes pointing straight forward, and your hands gripping the counter for balance.

2. Keep your back straight and your heels flat on the floor.

3. Slowly bend your knees, up to a 90-degree angle if comfortable (thighs will be horizontal), while pressing down on your little toes and keeping your knees over your feet as much as possible.

4. Straighten to your original position.

Try and get into the habit of doing a few sit-downs after you've been standing for more than 5 minutes. Not only will you get yourself into a great exercise routine, but you'll keep the blood moving in those legs!

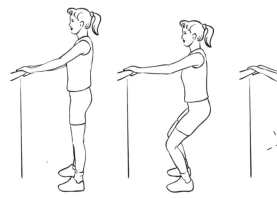

Sit-downs.

Heel-Ups

This exercise works your lower legs. You can make it a little harder by doing one leg at a time, wrapping your other foot around the ankle to be raised.

1. Place your feet on a block of wood or on a step so that your toes and the balls of your feet are supported but that your heels extend over the edge. Hold onto a counter or sturdy railing for balance.

2. Keeping your body straight and upright, let your heels sag as far below your toes as possible.

3. Raise up on the balls of your feet as far as you can, and then return to the starting position. Do this movement slowly and smoothly, and make sure your ankles do not roll outward.

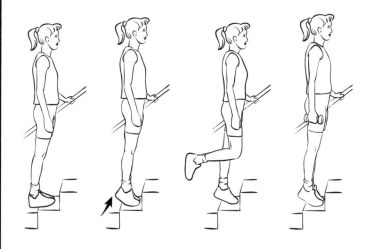

Heel-ups.

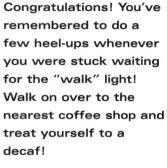
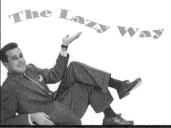

GET STRONG WHILE STAYING STILL

Another way that you can prod your bod is with isometric exercises. This kind of strength training challenges your muscles by forcing them to hold a contraction without moving. So you can get strong while staying still! The strength you gain from static contractions is limited to the angle at which you hold your joint. This means you will not develop strength throughout the full range of movement for the muscle (or muscle group) you are contracting. But it's still a great way to build muscle endurance, so give the next few exercises a try.

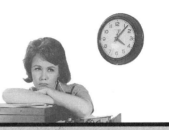

A COMPLETE WASTE OF TIME

The 3 Worst Ways to Do a Wall Sit:

1. Wearing high heels (or even just socks).

2. Leaning against a door (especially revolving ones).

3. Keeping your buttocks on the floor.

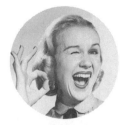

Leaning on the Wall

It won't take long for you to feel your thighs get warm when you do this exercise. It's a great one to help get your legs conditioned for downhill skiing.

1. Start by standing one and a half to two feet from the wall with your feet shoulder-width apart and your toes pointed straight ahead.

2. Lower yourself into a sitting position, with your back, knees, and feet forming a right angle (90 degrees), as if you were sitting on an invisible chair.

3. Stay in this position as long as possible. Return to standing.

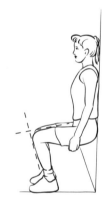

Leaning on the wall.

Lying Down Arches

This exercise will challenge your torso stabilization. It strengthens your buttocks, back, and thighs. Lying down arches are an effective isometric exercise, but they also work well if you add movement. Instead of holding the position, you can do several repetitions (raising up and then lowering back down).

1. Lie on your back with your arms straight out at your sides, with both knees bent and both feet flat on the floor.

2. Keeping your upper back on the floor, slowly raise your buttocks until there is an imaginary straight line from your shoulders to your knees. Don't arch your back.

3. Hold this position for a count of 30 or 60, and then slowly lower your pelvis back to the floor.

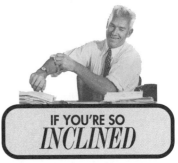

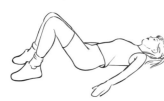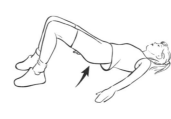

Lying down arches.

IF YOU'RE SO INCLINED

You can turn lying down arches into strength training in motion by doing a set of 12 to 15 repetitions. Instead of holding the contraction for a long time, just hold it for a few seconds, again and again and again.

If you spend a lot of time sitting in front of a computer, the lower back arches could become your best friend for improved lower back health. A few in the morning, and a few after work could make a world of difference!

Lower Back Arches

These arches are mainly for strengthening your lower back, but you'll feel them in your legs and buttocks, too. Keep your hips pressed down into the floor when you do this exercise.

1. Lie face down with your feet slightly apart and your arms stretched out in front of you.

2. Keeping your chin down, slowly lift your head, neck and chest three to six inches off the floor at the same time that you lift your feet and legs three to six inches off the floor. Be sure to keep your abdominal muscles tightened and your hips pressed into the floor.

3. Hold this position as long as possible, and then return to the starting position.

Lower back arches.

ADD SOME STRENGTH TO A STROLL IN THE PARK

Now that you have some effective exercises that use your body for resistance, you can get in strength training anywhere you take it. One of the best places to add some strength is outdoors, in your neighborhood or at a park. Try these moves the next time you take a stroll:

- Do your push-ups leaning on the back of a park bench.
- Swing on the monkey bars.
- Do your dips on a bench or car bumper. (Instead of moving your elbows out to the sides, point them behind you as you bend your arms.)
- Take off your shoes and do walking kneel-downs (lunges) in the sand.
- Grab onto a pole and do your sit-downs (squats) or heel-ups (calf raises).

If you want to get a complete workout in 15 minutes, go for a stroll to warm up and then alternate the following aerobic activities with the preceding strength exercises. Do any of these aerobic moves for 2 minutes before each strength move:

- Jumping jacks
- Skipping
- Scooting
- Jogging in place
- Step-ups
- Speed skating (in place)

Congratulations! You did some strength training! Now it's time to rest your muscles. Don't even think about lifting a weight for at least 48 hours.

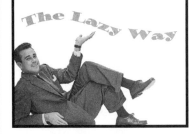

The Lazy Way

Getting Time on Your Side

	The Old Way	The Lazy Way
Strength training your upper body	20 minutes	6 to 8 minutes
Strength training your lower body	20 minutes	6 to 8 minutes
Getting in a complete workout	60 minutes	15 minutes
Getting your equipment together	10 minutes	No time at all!
Finding a place to work out	30 minutes	You're there!
Feeling pain	Often	Never again!

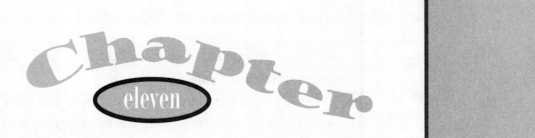

A Little Weight Goes a Long Way

What do an ounce of courage, a few kind words, and a dollop of horseradish have in common with a pair of dumbbells? Not much really except that you don't need a lot of them to notice a big difference. That's how it is with dumbbells—a little weight goes a long way!

When you add weights to your strength training routine, you increase the workload on your muscles. They respond by growing stronger and more shapely. Of course, they'll do this better if you let them rest after you work them. The key thing is you never have to overwork them. All you need to do is add a little weight, and this chapter will show you how.

GETTING FIRM WITHOUT THE SQUIRM

The simplest way to add weight to your workout (besides using your body) is with dumbbells and ankle weights. That way, you don't have to worry about getting tangled in cables or roller pads. You don't have to wonder whether you are sitting too low or too high on a chrome fixture, and you don't

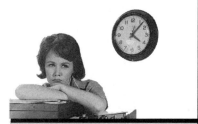

need to be concerned that anything other than your own muscles is stabilizing your body for you.

When you strength train with dumbbells and ankle weights, you have the freedom to work in every plane of movement. The only adjustment you need to make is to securely fasten the straps of your ankle weights. You'll also get the added benefit of improving your balance and coordination when you stabilize your body. There's no doubt that using these simple weights will get you firm without the squirm!

MOVES FOR YOUR UPPER BODY

There are lots of strengthening moves using dumbbells for your upper body. Some of them work a group of muscles; others target a specific muscle. Either way, they are all pretty simple and very effective. The following sections describe some of the best ones.

Lying Down Press-Ups

These press-ups work your chest and the front of your shoulders. They are a much better version of increasing your bust than holding your arms out in front of you and squeezing your palms together.

1. Grasp two dumbbells and lie on your back on a flat bench, with your knees bent and your feet flat on the bench. Hold the dumbbells at your sides by your chest.

2. While looking up at the ceiling, slowly raise the dumbbells over your chest (over nipple line) until they come together. Your elbows should be slightly bent.

3. Slowly bring the dumbbells down. Repeat for the desired number of repetitions.

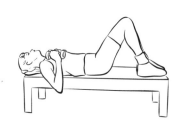 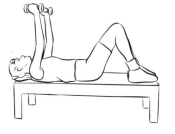

Lying down press-ups.

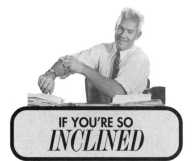

IF YOU'RE SO
INCLINED

You must, you must, you must increase your bust!! If you get tired of the same old chest routine, try doings some lying down press-ups with dumbbells. They will uplift you in no time!

Bending Over Pulls

This move resembles starting a lawn mower (the kind with a cord, not a switch). It will strengthen your upper back and arm muscles and stretch your chest.

1. Stand to the right of a stable chair, with a weight in your right hand.

2. Place your left knee on the chair, extending the leg back about 18 inches to the rear and keep both knees bent.

3. Bend over from the hips, and place your left palm on the chair seat for support and to brace your torso, keeping your left elbow slightly bent.

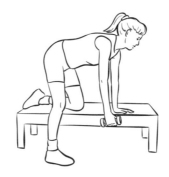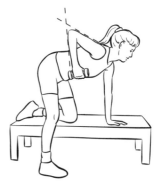

Bending over pulls.

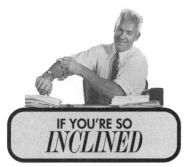

IF YOU'RE SO
INCLINED

Waiting for water to boil? do a few Bending Over Pulls while you're stuck in the kitchen with nothing to do!

4. Hold the dumbbell in your right hand with the palm facing your body's midline. The weight should be level with the chair. Then slowly pull the weight up until it lightly touches the side of your rib cage, pulling your left shoulder blade back at the top of the movement.

5. Slowly lower the dumbbell back down to the starting position and repeat 12 to 15 times.

6. Repeat this exercise with the weight in your left hand and your right knee on the chair.

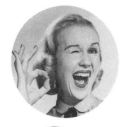

QUICK 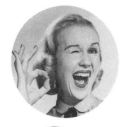 PAINLESS

All you need for bending over pulls is yourself, a chair, and a weight...what could be easier? Next time you're in the kitchen, grab an economy size can of soup (you know, the "Family Size"), a chair, and you're off!

Lying Down Arm Raises

This exercise is great because it always feels good to lie on your side. This exercise strengthens your shoulders, especially the back part of them.

1. Lie on your side with your legs straight and your top arm stretched out in front of you.

2. Hold a light weight with your top hand and slowly raise your straight arm toward the ceiling. Do not go beyond your body's midline.

3. Slowly bring your arm back down.

4. Repeat for the desired number of repetitions, and then turn onto your other side and lift the other arm.

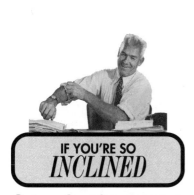

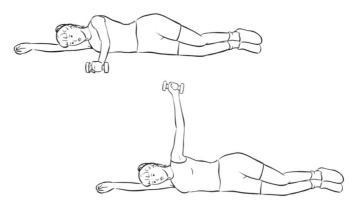

Lying down arm raises.

Arm Swings

This exercise also strengthens your shoulders, emphasizing the rotator cuff. If you swing a racket, bat, or golf club, you definitely want to do this one.

1. Stand up straight, holding a dumbbell on your right side. Your arm should be bent at the elbow to form a right angle.

2. Keeping your right elbow next to your side, start moving your arm outwards. Your forearm should stay parallel to the floor.

3. Rotate your right arm as far as it will go without your elbow leaving your side.

4. Bring your arm slowly back to the starting position and repeat 10 to 12 times.

5. Repeat the same process with your left arm.

YOU'LL THANK YOURSELF LATER

Strengthen your shoulders by doing some arm swings (for rotators). That way, you'll save yourself from striking out on your next swing!

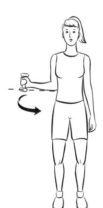

Arm swings.

When doing curl-ups for the first time, start off with minimal weight. As you get used to the exercise, you can use some more weight. It won't do anyone any good if you pull your muscles by overdoing it before you've even gotten started!

Curl-Ups

Are you ready for some buffed biceps? Then this is the exercise for you! But be careful not to overdo them, or Popeye might get jealous.

1. Stand or sit erect, with your elbows pulled into your sides.

2. Grasp the weights with your hands, palms facing upward.

3. Keeping your elbows at your sides, bend your arms and pull the weights up to your shoulders.

4. Slowly return to the starting position.

5. Repeat for the desired number of repetitions.

You can also alternate arms for this exercise. Make sure your arms come back down all the way.

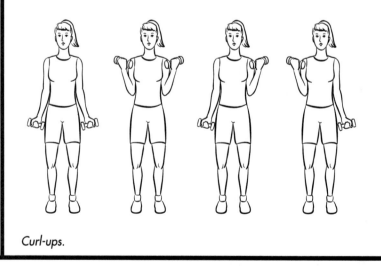

Curl-ups.

Back Scratchers

If you want to stop your arms from flapping, add this exercise to your routine. It does wonders for firming up the backs of your arms.

1. Standing or seated erect, grasp one weight with both hands, palms up, and bring your arms straight up overhead.

2. Hold the dumbbell vertically, with the thumb and index finger of each hand, with one hand below the other.

3. Bend your elbows, lowering the weight behind your head.

4. Straighten your elbows, pushing the weight up over-head again.

5. Keep your arms close to your ears throughout this exercise.

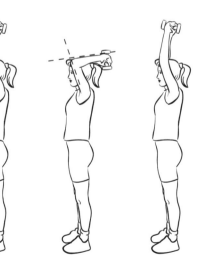

Back scratchers.

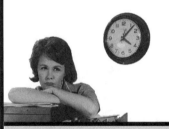

A COMPLETE WASTE OF TIME

The 3 Worst Things to Do for Flappy Arms:

1. Ignore them.

2. Hide them.

3. Yell at them.

MOVES FOR YOUR LOWER BODY

It's a little hard to lift a dumbbell with your foot, so you'll want to keep them in your hands (even when you work your legs). Another alternative is wearing ankle weights. The following exercises will show you how to use both.

Step-Ups, Kneel-Downs, and Heel-Ups with More Than Your Body Weight

When you are ready for a bigger challenge, add a little weight to your kneel-downs, step-ups, and heel-ups. Just follow the directions given in Chapter 10 for these moves, but hold a couple of dumbbells at your sides. When you do heel-ups, you'll need one hand to balance you, so hold a dumbbell in the other hand, which should correspond to the foot being worked.

A SIMPLE SET WITH SUPER RESULTS

You can do this simple, quick, all-in-one set when you have a pair of light weights and 10 minutes to spare. It works your upper and lower body; plus it raises your heart rate. The wonderful thing about this set is that it challenges your muscles in the different planes of movement (front, side, and diagonal). This range of movement will help increase your coordination and flexibility.

If you don't have a pair of dumbbells, you can use soup cans, water bottles filled with sand, or even a pair of heavy shoes (great for when you're in a hotel room). Just pick up what you can find and get ready for a simple workout that consists of three sets with three parts.

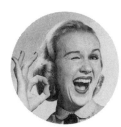

QUICK ☜☞ PAINLESS

Dumbbells aren't just for your upper body. You can also use them to work your legs. All you have to do is hold them at your sides when you do step-ups, heel-ups, or kneel-downs.

Set One

Hold dumbbells at your shoulders with arms bent. Stand up straight with abdominals pulled in.

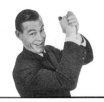

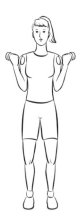

Starting position for set one.

YOU'LL THANK YOURSELF LATER

If you know you won't have any access to dumbbells when traveling, buy a couple bottles of water and use them instead. You can drink them after you've done your simple, super set.

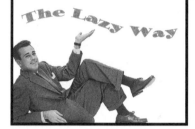

Congratulations! You can see some definition in your arms now. Go out and buy yourself something sleeveless.

The Lazy Way

In the first part of this set (Part A), you are working on your arms, back and abdominals:

1. Lift your right arm straight up over your head.

2. Bring your right arm down to the starting position and then lift your left arm. Alternate arms three to five times.

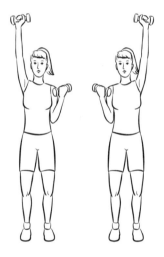

Part A of set one.

In the second part of this set (Part B), you are working on your arms, chest and abdominals:

1. Lift your right arm over your head in the form of a *c*. Palms should face the midline of your body.

2. Bring down your right arm to the starting position and then lift your left arm. Alternate arms three to five times.

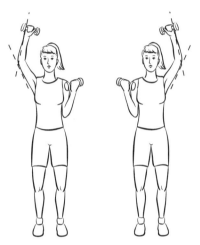

Part B of set one.

In the third part of this set (Part C), you are working on your arms, chest, abdominals and back:

1. Lift your right arm in front of your face and diagonally up past your forehead. Your palms should face your forehead. Your hips should turn with your arms.

2. Bring down your right arm to the starting position and then lift your left arm. Alternate arms three to five times.

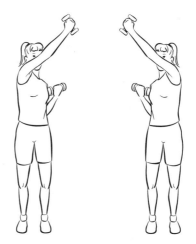

Part C of set one.

Set Two

Hold the dumbbells down at your sides. Stand up straight with abdominals pulled in. Arms should be straight with a slight bend at elbows for this set. Although you will be working on the same sets of muscles as you did in the first set, by straightening out your arms (with respect to the first set of exercises) you will be increasing the resistance to your muscles, and also incorporating more muscle groups.

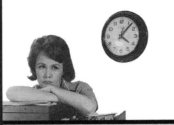

A COMPLETE WASTE OF TIME

The 3 Worst Ways to Use Dumbbells:

1. As a doorstop.

2. As a paperweight.

3. As a volleyball.

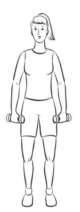

Starting position for set two.

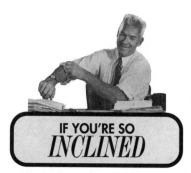

Putting away the groceries? Do this exercise with your soup cans and kill two birds with one stone!

Part A of set two:

1. Lift your right arm straight up over your head.

2. Bring down your right arm to the starting position and then lift your left arm. Alternate arms three to five times.

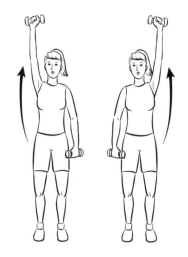

Part A of set two.

Part B of set two:

1. Lift your right arm over your head in the form of a c. Palms should face the midline of your body.

2. Bring down your right arm to the starting position and then lift your left arm. Alternate arms three to five times.

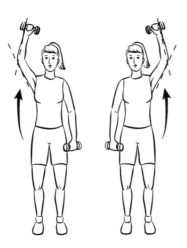

Part B of set two.

Part C of set two:

1. Lift your right arm in front of your face and diagonally up past your forehead. Your palms should face your forehead.

2. Bring down your right arm to the starting position and then lift your left arm. Alternate arms three to five times.

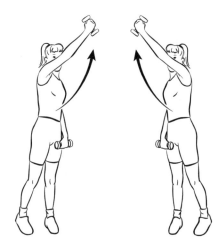

Part C of set two.

QUICK 🔲 PAINLESS

Go 3-D! When you strength train, move your body in different planes (front, side, diagonal). This variety will increase your balance, coordination, and flexibility.

Set Three

In this set, arm movements are combined with lunges. Not only does this mean that you will be incorporating the lower body into the exercises from the first two sets, but it also means you will be giving yourself more of a total body workout.

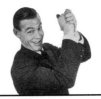

Remember: Always warm up with same stretches before you start exercising! Your muscles will thank you!

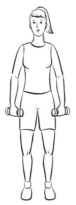

Starting position for set three.

Part A of set three:

1. Start with the dumbbells held down at your sides and feet slightly apart and facing forward. Do a forward lunge, taking the dumbbells down to the floor by your front foot.

2. Move your front leg back to starting position, lifting the dumbbells over your head at the same time.

3. Repeat the forward lunge with the other leg, bringing dumbbells down to the floor again as you move forward. Alternate legs three to five times.

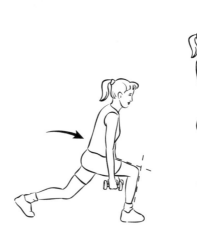

Part A of set three.

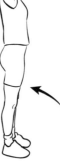

Part B of set three:

1. Start with dumbbells held down at your sides and your feet slightly apart and facing forward. Do a side lunge (still facing forward), taking the dumbbells down to the floor by your bent leg.

2. Move your leg back to its starting position, lifting the dumbbells over your head at the same time.

3. Repeat the side lunge with the other leg, bringing dumbbells down to floor again as you move sideways. Alternate legs three to five times.

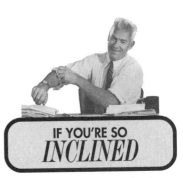

IF YOU'RE SO
INCLINED

Try doing these exercises in front of a mirror so you can keep an eye on your form.

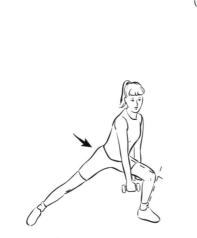

Part B of set three.

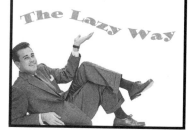
Part C of set three:

1. Pivot to a 45-degree angle behind you (if you were facing 12 o'clock, pivot to 4 o'clock), taking dumbbells down to the floor by your front foot.

2. Pivot back to the starting position (12 o'clock), lifting the dumbbells over your head at the same time.

3. Repeat the diagonal lunge with the other leg, bringing dumbbells down to the floor again as you pivot backwards.

Once you've completed all of the sets and their parts, go ahead and repeat this cycle one or two more times.

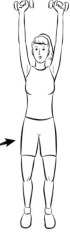
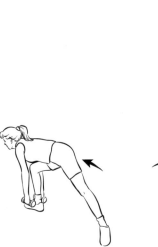

Part C of set three.

Getting Time on Your Side

	The Old Way	The Lazy Way
Working out your arms with dumbbells	15 minutes	6 minutes
Working out your chest with dumbbells	12 minutes	4 minutes
Working out your back with dumbbells	16 minutes	4 minutes
Working out your right leg with dumbbells	15 minutes	8 minutes
Working out your left leg with dumbbells	12 minutes	5 minutes
Working out your whole body with dumbbells	58 minutes	22 minutes

Use Some Rubber to Melt the Blubber

You've shied away from strength training, and who wouldn't? It seems so heavy-duty! The machines in the gym look like torture contraptions, and the risk of breaking a nail while using dumbbells has got to be above average. You can set those fears aside by strength training with some rubber.

Adding some rubber to your workout will challenge your body without you having to lift a weight. You'll still build strong muscles, which is great because the more muscle you have, the more fat you'll burn. So you see, using some rubber really can melt the blubber! This chapter shows you how to spring into action using rubber bands and balls, and provides lots of simple exercises to choose from.

GREAT TOOLS FOR SHAPING UP ACCORDING TO LAZY WAY RULES

Rubber bands and balls are wonderful strength training tools, especially for shaping up according to *The Lazy Way* rules. They are lightweight and convenient, which makes them a great choice for traveling. They are challenging for all fitness levels; you can make your workout harder by shortening the band or changing your position on the ball. Last, but not least, they're fun! Let's see how each one works.

Strike Up the Band

A band of rubber (including elastic tubing) works your muscles by providing resistance. Depending on which muscles you want to work, you can hold or tie it around any part of your body, or you can wrap it around poles or banisters. The beauty of the band is that it offers you a complete workout and then you can put it away in a drawer.

To get the most out of your rubber band workout, adhere to these band basics:

- Bands come in a variety of resistances; the thicker the band, the harder the workout.

- If you need to tie the band, make a simple square knot and then pull on the band to make sure the knot is secure, but not too tight. Keep your loop 8 to 10 inches in diameter.

- Untie and flatten your band after use and before storing.

- You can use a normal grip to hold the ends of the band or you can wrap it around your hands (always remove large rings). If the band hurts your hands, wear workout gloves.

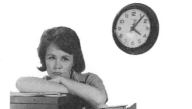

A COMPLETE WASTE OF TIME

The 3 Worst Ways to Use an Exercise Band:

1. As a tie.
2. As a scarf.
3. As a sweat band.

- Before you begin each exercise, make sure the band is securely in place. Adjust the position of the band if a motion bothers your joints.

- Avoid pulling the band toward your face or eyes.

- Do not store your band in direct sunlight. Sprinkle it with talcum powder every now and then to freshen it up and prevent the rubber from sticking.

- A band should last about four to five months. Replace it with a new one as soon as you notice a hole or tear.

Have a Ball

Ball exercises are great for improving your balance, posture, coordination, and strength. The beauty of the ball is that its surface is unstable. This instability constantly challenges you to maintain good posture and stay in balance throughout each movement. Your whole body will end up getting stronger and more stable, especially your midsection (lower back and abdominals).

Here are a few things you need to know before you get the ball rolling:

- Stability balls come in all sizes and colors, and they are fairly inexpensive. (See the section about shaping up your home gym in Appendix A—specifically "Resist-A-Ball" for ordering information.)

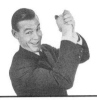

YOU'LL THANK YOURSELF LATER

Be sure to choose the right color when buying an exercise band. Don't go for what will look good with your fitness outfit, but rather what will give you the proper resistance. Pink is the least resistant; green is low to medium; purple is medium; gray is greatest.

- Choose the right size ball for your height. When sitting on the ball, with feet flat, the hips and knees should form a 90-degree angle. Use these guidelines for determining appropriate ball size:

Height	Ball Size
Less than 5 feet tall	17-inch ball
5'0" to 5'7"	21-inch ball
5'8" to 6'2"	25-inch ball
6'3" and over	29-inch ball

- For proper inflation, see the instructions that come with the ball. Be careful not to overinflate the ball, especially if you are using an air compressor. A fully inflated or firm ball has less contact area and moves more quickly (making it harder to maintain balance); an underinflated ball has greater contact area and moves more slowly (making it easier to maintain your balance).

- If you want to travel with your ball, just deflate it for packing and inflate it with your blow dryer (using the appropriate nozzle adapter) when you're ready to exercise.

- The farther away the ball is from your body, the more challenging the exercise. Closing your eyes also increases the difficulty of the exercise.

- When you're at home, leave the ball out to encourage you and your family to exercise, stretch, and play with it.

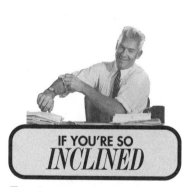

IF YOU'RE SO
INCLINED

To give yourself an extra challenge with your ball exercises, just add more air. The firmer the ball, the faster it will move, and the harder it will be to stay balanced.

ELASTIC MOVES FOR YOUR UPPER BODY

It doesn't take much to feel your muscles work against an exercise band. Do a set or two of 8 to 10 repetitions. You should feel the tension with every repetition, and the last rep should be so challenging that you can't do another one with good form. When the reps get easy, it's time to shorten the band or use a thicker one.

Congratulations! You've graduated to a thicker and shorter band! Treat yourself to a day at the beach!

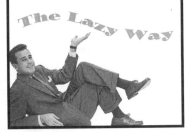

The Lazy Way

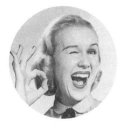

 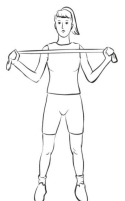
Pull-Downs

This exercise feels great on the back. It will tone up the muscles along the sides of your back into the waist.

1. Stand or sit up straight and extend your arms straight in front of you, holding the elastic tubing at forehead level. Hands should be a little less than a foot apart from each other.

2. Pull the band down toward your chest, squeezing your shoulder blades together. The distance between your hands will widen as your arms come down.

3. Return to your starting position and repeat the movement 10 to 15 times.

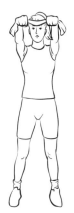
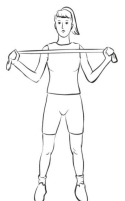

Pull-downs.

Sitting Down Pulls

This exercise will strengthen your upper back and help improve your upper body posture. It's a great one for those of you who tend to be round-shouldered.

1. Sit on the floor with your legs out in front of you, keeping your back straight and abdominals pulled in.

2. Wrap the elastic tubing around your feet and hold the ends of the tubing in each hand, with your arms extended in front of you.

3. With your knees slightly bent, slowly pull your arms toward your waist, pushing your chest out and squeezing your shoulder blades together. Keep your abdominals tight so that your lower back doesn't arch.

4. Slowly return to the starting position and repeat the movement for the desired number of times.

5. You can make this exercise harder by shortening the length of elastic tubing (wrap more of it around your hand).

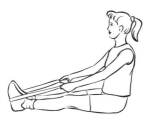 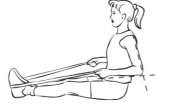

Sitting down pulls.

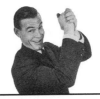

YOU'LL THANK YOURSELF LATER

Posture, posture, posture! By working on it now, you'll be helping yourself out in a way that will last the rest of your life—be good to your back!

Back Scratchers with a Band

Back scratchers are a sure hit for toning the back of your arms. You can make this exercise a little harder by standing on one end of the band instead of holding it behind you at your waist.

1. Start with your feet apart, right foot in front of the left and knees slightly bent.

2. Hold a band with your left hand behind your back, elbow bent at the small of your back with thumb pointing up.

3. Loosely wrap the other end of the band around your right hand and bring it behind your head, elbow bent and thumb pointing down. You should feel tension at both ends of the band.

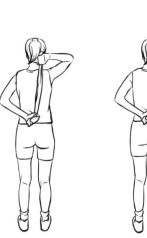

Back scratchers with a band.

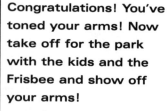
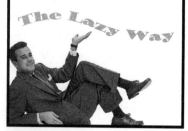

4. Without changing your body position, push your right hand upwards to the ceiling. Keep your arm directly above your shoulder and in line with your right ear throughout the exercise.

5. Slowly release to the start position and repeat the movement for the desired number of repetitions.

6. Change sides to work the back of the other arm.

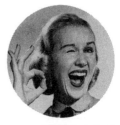

QUICK **☐☐** *PAINLESS*

Need to exercise but don't want to miss your favorite show on TV? Do both at the same time!

ELASTIC MOVES FOR YOUR LOWER BODY

You'll need to tie the ends of the band together for most leg exercises (follow the instructions given earlier in this chapter). The following three simple band exercises will work your legs from hip to toe.

Rocking Horse

The rocking horse strengthens your buttocks and thighs and challenges your balance. It's okay to hold onto a counter for support if you need to.

1. Tie the ends of the band together and loop the band around the arches of both feet. You should feel a slight tension in the band. If not, retie it to make the loop smaller.

2. Stand up straight with abs pulled in and feet apart, with the right foot slightly in front of the left.

3. Keeping your pelvis in a neutral position, lift your right knee to hip height.

4. Step onto your right foot and, keeping your knee slightly bent, straighten your left leg behind you until you feel your buttocks contract. Don't lean forward or backward.

5. Repeat the sequence for desired amount of repetitions and then switch legs.

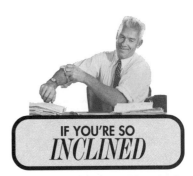

IF YOU'RE SO
INCLINED

It's ok to start off a balancing act with a little extra support—as you strengthen your muscles, you'll find you don't need that extra help any more!

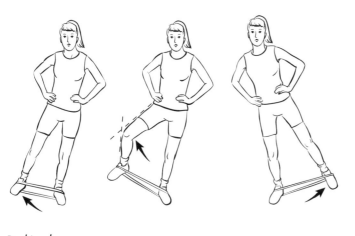

Rocking horse.

Outer Thigh Pulls

You'll be feeling these pulls right about where those sad-dlebags hang. Be sure to keep your hips pressed into the floor when doing this exercise.

1. Tie the ends of the band together and loop it around your ankles. Lie on your stomach and rest your forehead on your hands.

2. Keeping your right leg still, pull your left one out to the side as far as you can. Your hips and toes should stay in contact with the floor throughout this exercise.

3. Relax the leg back to the starting position and repeat the exercise for the desired number of repetitions.

4. Switch legs.

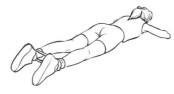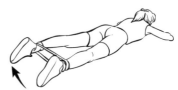

Outer thigh pulls.

Congratulations! You've done Outer Thigh Pulls for a week! Go out dancing with your favorite person and show off those legs!

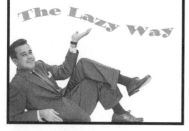

Point and Flex

This exercise is for your lower legs. It's a great one for those of you who have weak ankles or shins. You can do it sitting up or reclining on your shoulders.

1. Sit on the floor with your left leg out in front of you and your right leg bent at the knee with the foot flat on the floor.

2. Wrap the band around your left foot and hold the ends in each hand with your arms extended in front of you.

3. Keeping the tension on the band, slowly point and flex your left foot, working as hard as possible against the resistance of the band. Repeat 15 to 20 times.

4. Switch legs.

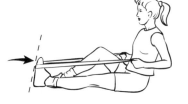

Point and flex.

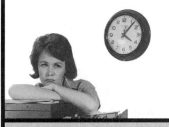

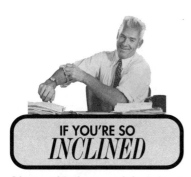

IF YOU'RE SO
INCLINED

Not playing with your tennis balls too much during the winter months? Here's a way to use them: Place a ball between your knees when you do your lying down arches. You'll feel it in your inner thighs.

PLAY BALL!

Just sitting on a stability ball can be an exercise. It teaches you to find your neutral position (not too arched or too flat in the back, but somewhere in between). By adding a little movement, you can create lots of exercises on the ball. Here are some effective ones for increasing your core strength.

Lying Down Walk-Out

This exercise will strengthen your arm and shoulder muscles and improve your balance reactions.

1. Place yourself over the ball, resting on your hands and knees (stomach is on top of the ball).

2. Keeping head down and abs pulled in, start walking your arms out until the ball is under your thighs. Don't let your abdominals sag.

3. Walk your arms back towards ball to start position. Repeat a few more times. Stop when you can't keep the proper form.

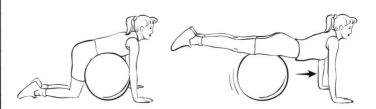

Lying down walk-out.

Trunk Raises

Trunk raises will strengthen your back, neck, and arm muscles. This exercise feels so good that you can do as many reps as you like.

1. Lie with your abdomen on the ball and your body weight resting on your hands and balls of your feet. Your legs are extended behind you with knees slightly bent.

2. Slowly and smoothly raise your trunk and arms up. Your arms are straight in front of you and your head should be aligned between them. Press hips into the ball as you raise up.

3. Slowly lower yourself down to start position and repeat for the desired number of repetitions.

Trunk raises.

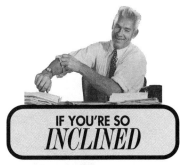

IF YOU'RE SO
INCLINED

Try listening to a little slow music when doing trunk raises and see if you can time the exercise to the music. You'll end up concentrating on the timing so much that you might just forget you're exercising!

Sit Down to Lying Down Arch with Ball

This exercise stretches and strengthens your hip and leg muscles. It also challenges your torso to stabilize itself.

1. Sit on the floor with feet flat, knees bent, and back leaning against the ball. Hands can stay on your hips.

2. Lift your hips up, resting your shoulders and head on the ball. Your back should be parallel to the floor, with your knees at a 90-degree angle. Hold this position for a count of 30.

3. Lower yourself back to the start position and repeat the exercise a few more times. Stop when you lose form.

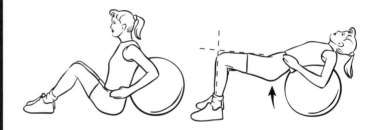

Sit down to lying down arch with ball.

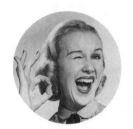

QUICK 🔟 PAINLESS

Ball Rolls Up the Wall

These ball rolls will strengthen your thighs and hips. They will also increase your range of motion. You need a wall for this exercise.

1. Lie on your back a couple of feet away from a wall, with your arms relaxed at your sides. Your left leg is bent at the knee with the left foot flat on the floor (toes can touch the wall). Your right leg is bent at a 45-degree angle, with the knee facing forward and your right foot on the ball, which is against the wall.

2. Extend your right leg, rolling the ball upwards along the wall. Then roll the ball back down to the starting position. Repeat this exercise for the desired number of repetitions.

3. Switch legs.

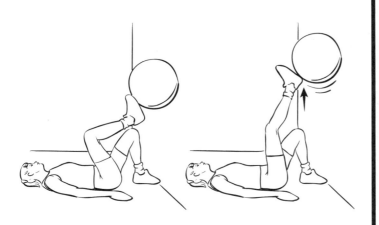

Ball rolls up the wall.

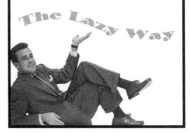

Congratulations! You got that ball up the wall! Now take your favorite pooch out for a walk and let him chase the ball for a while!

Getting Time on Your Side

	The Old Way	The Lazy Way
Strength training your upper body with the band	20 minutes	8 minutes
Strength training your lower body with the band	20 minutes	10 minutes
Strength training your upper body with the ball	20 minutes	8 minutes
Strength training your lower body with the ball	20 minutes	8 minutes
Putting away your equipment	5 minutes	30 seconds
Feeling good while you work out	Impossible!	Always!

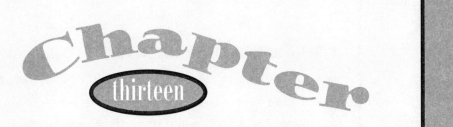

thirteen

Trade Your Rolls for Ripples

You are proud of the fact that you're not obsessed about your middle. Heck, it has even worked to your advantage; while everyone else has been torturing themselves to get a "six-pack," you've been able to acquire a keg. Unfortunately, you have discovered that, in some cases, more isn't necessarily better. So how can you trade your rolls for ripples without having to chug—oops! I meant tug—too hard?

All you have to do is shape up your middle *The Lazy Way!* That means you can throw away all of your belly-buster gadgets and forget about doing hundreds of sit-ups. I'll show you what's necessary to melt down your middle and will give you some easy and effective exercises to flatten your stomach. Plus, you'll see why what's good for the front is great for the back.

YOUR MIDDLE MELTDOWN

So if you don't have to do hundreds of sit-ups, just what does it take to melt the fat around your middle? You have to huff and puff to lose the fluff. Remember, aerobic exercise is what burns the fat (even your belly). Abdominal crunches also have a place in slimming down your middle, but only if they are done correctly. Keep these pointers in mind while trying to tighten your tummy:

- Forget about using abdominal machines. The most effective (not to mention convenient) way to work your abs is on the floor. Just follow the exercises given in this chapter.

- Get rid of the notion that you have to work your middle every single day. Abdominal exercises can be done as little as four times per week, spread out over as many days as possible.

- Don't forget the importance of eating well and exercising (aerobically) regularly. These foundations are required for your middle meltdown.

- Be sure to drink plenty of water, especially if you are experiencing water retention (swollen abdomen). Drinking water will help release stored fluid and get rid of excess sodium.

- Essentially, every exercise you do includes working your abs. Keep your tummy tucked in for whatever exercise you are doing. This rule goes for when you are standing, sitting, kneeling, or lying down.

QUICK ⏲ *PAINLESS*

Get a grip on those love handles! If you are carrying fat around your middle, the best way to get it off is with aerobic exercise, not stomach crunches.

WHAT'S GOOD FOR THE FRONT IS GREAT FOR THE BACK

Working your abs isn't just for looks. Abs play an important role in stabilizing your torso and supporting your lower back. Your abs are the core of your body's structural system. When you do what's good for your front, you definitely help your back. Here are some more ways you can protect your back.

No More Bellyaching About Backaches

If you don't have any back pain, you probably know somebody who does. This common problem is often caused by weak abdominals, poor posture, too much sitting, improper lifting, and inadequate flexibility. The good news is that those are all things you can change. Follow these tips and you won't have to bellyache about backaches.

- Never bend and twist your back at the same time; move your feet to turn your body.

- Always assume good posture (Chapter 14 will show you how).

- Stretch your legs often. Tight hamstrings and hip flexors can pull on your back.

- Keep objects close to your body when lifting or carrying.

- If something is too heavy to lift comfortably, get help.

- When sitting, try to keep your knees lower than your hips.

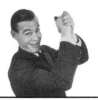

YOU'LL THANK YOURSELF LATER

Think twice before doing the twist! Train yourself to move your feet to turn your body. That way, the next time you twist your body, you won't tweak your back.

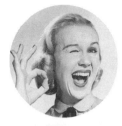

- Don't let back braces or weight belts be a substitute for strong abdominal and buttock muscles.

- Many strength and flexibility exercises can help you get your back in shape. They include lower back arches (Chapter 10, p. 110), lying down arches (Chapter 10, p. 109), back leg looseners (Chapter 16, p. 202), hip unflexors (Chapter 16, p. 204), knee huggers (Chapter 16, p. 200), upper back unbinders (Chapter 16, p. 197), plop-overs (Chapter 16, p. 201), up and down arches (Chapter 16, p. 206), lying down liberators (Chapter 16, p. 208), back releasers (Chapter 16, p. 207), spinal stabilizers (Chapter 15, p. 180), and all of the abdominal exercises in this chapter.

Don't Bend Over Backwards

Sometimes we don't realize how much we bend over until we get hurt and can't do it anymore. Bending your body is such a common occurrence that it's important to make sure you do it correctly. Here's the correct way to pick up an object from the ground:

1. Keep your feet at least shoulder-width apart to provide a base of support. It's ok to point your feet out.

2. As you squat, extend your buttocks as far backward as you can to maintain an arch in your lower back. Keep your heels on the floor and your knees over your feet.

3. Place your hands on the object, and using your leg muscles to power the lift, stand up. Remember to keep the object as close to you as possible and keep your back straight as you lift.

4. If you need to raise your arms over your head, tuck your buttocks in and tighten your abs. Don't let your back arch.

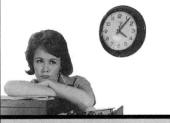

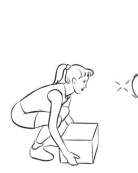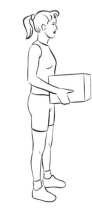

The proper way to lift.

A COMPLETE WASTE OF TIME

The 3 Worst Ways to Pick Up an Object:

1. With straight legs.
2. When your hands are full.
3. Wearing stilts.

SIMPLE MOVES TO KEEP YOUR STOMACH SLEEK AND FLAT

Abdominal crunches are much easier to do than you may think. First of all, you get to do them lying down. Next, you do each exercise slowly and smoothly. Finally, you don't have to do a lot of them. Begin with 10 repetitions of each exercise and gradually work up to 25 or more. That's all folks!

Pull-Ins

This exercise will teach you how to breathe properly when working your abdominals. It's a great one to do at the beginning of your ab routine.

1. Lie on your back with your knees bent and your feet flat on the floor (alternately, you can have your legs on a chair and your knees at right angles).

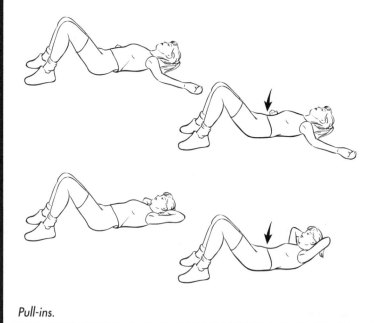

Pull-ins.

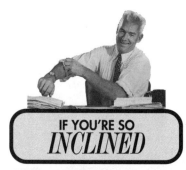

2. Inhale deeply, allowing your middle to expand.

3. Slowly exhale and at the same time tilt your hips upward, pressing your back down onto the floor. Don't let your hips come off the floor.

4. Contract your abdomen, pulling your belly button closer to your spine while exhaling all of the air in your lungs. It's important to keep your belly flat and force all the air out because this is what works the deepest layers of your abs.

5. Relax and breathe in. Repeat the exercise.

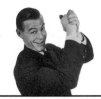

YOU'LL THANK YOURSELF LATER

If your pouch is making you feel like a kangaroo, go ahead and jump into a girdle. You'll get a flat tummy without a lot of effort (although that depends on how hard it is to put on the girdle).

Pull In and Ups

This exercise is just like a pull-in except you bring your upper torso off the ground at the same time. It targets the front abdominal muscles (transverse).

1. Lie on your back with your knees bent, and your feet flat on the floor about shoulder-width apart. Cup your hands under your head. Alternately, you can cross your hands over your chest and you can have your legs on a chair with your knees at right angles.

2. Slowly raise your upper torso off the ground. Don't pull on your neck, keep it in line with your trunk by keeping your elbows back.

3. Do the reverse curl procedure (step number 4 in the preceding pull-in exercise) simultaneously as you raise up. Exhale as you exert upward; inhale as you come down and relax. During this exercise your upper and lower body are being squeezed upward while you try to keep your belly button close to the ground.

4. For a more advanced version of this exercise, keep your arms outstretched above your head.

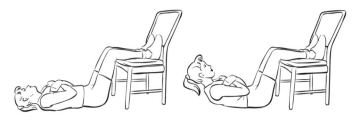

Pull in and ups (with variation).

Look for ways to add your own variations to these exercises, even if all you do is put the moves to music. Giving yourself a little variety will make the time pass faster!

Slide-Ups

Slide-ups emphasize the abdominal muscles that wrap around the side of your body (obliques). They're just a pull in and up with a slight twist.

1. Lie on your back with your knees bent and your feet about shoulder-width apart.

2. Cup your left hand under your head. Place your right hand across and onto the outer part of your left thigh.

3. Keeping both hips on the ground, contract your abdomen and slide your right hand upward along your left thigh.

4. Hold this for a count of five.

5. Exhale as you contract and raise your hand; inhale as you come down and relax.

6. Repeat the mirror image of this, placing your left hand on your right thigh.

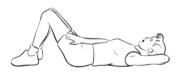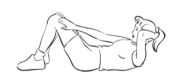

Slide-ups.

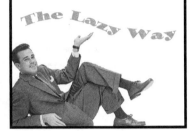

Congratulations! You've taken an inch off of your waist! Try tucking your blouse in and wearing a snazzy belt.

The Lazy Way

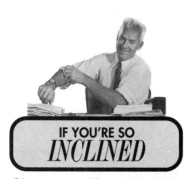

Trunk Turns

This exercise is very challenging. You need to have strong abs and no back problems to tackle this one.

1. Lie on your back, arms outstretched to the sides (your arms and body forming a letter T), palms on the floor, and hips and knees bent at right angles. Keep your shoulders on the ground throughout the exercise.

2. Keeping your knees together, slowly lower your legs to the right side of your body.

3. Smoothly raise your legs back up to the starting position and then lower them on the other side. Repeat the exercise.

4. Over time, gradually straighten your legs as you do the trunk turns.

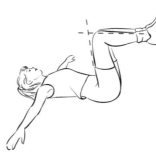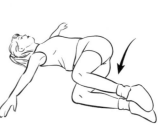

Trunk turns.

INSTEAD OF A THRUST, GO FOR A TILT

Even though abdominal crunches are most effective when you are lying down, it doesn't mean you can't work them while you're standing or sitting. You just need to give yourself a little tilt. Here's how:

1. Stand or sit up straight in your chair.

2. Breathe in, filling up your diaphragm (your middle should expand).

3. Forcefully blow all of your air out, pulling your belly button into your spine. If you are doing this correctly, it will make your hips tilt up slightly.

4. Repeat this breathing in and out process 10 to 20 times.

These tilts will not only help you improve your posture, they'll keep your tummy tucked. Make sure you incorporate them into your day. Here are a few suggestions to help you start a tilting routine:

▪ In your car, tilt at every red light.

▪ In the grocery store, tilt whenever you wait at the deli counter.

▪ At your desk, tilt whenever you turn on your computer.

▪ In a meeting, tilt whenever it gets boring.

▪ While watching TV, tilt during the first commercial of each break.

▪ In an airplane, tilt as you fasten your seat belt.

YOU'LL THANK YOURSELF LATER

The next time you're driving and the signal light turns yellow, don't rush to go through it. Instead, stop and do your tilts while you wait for the light to change.

Getting Time on Your Side

	The Old Way	The Lazy Way
Using the ab roller	15 minutes	0 minutes
Sitting and twisting	3 minutes	0 minutes
Doing abdominal crunches	Every day of the week	4 days a week
Getting through your ab routine	20 minutes	5 to 7 minutes
Working your sides	6 minutes	2 minutes
Work time lost from back pain	Days	None

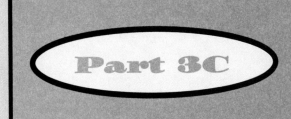

Part 3C

Your Flexibility: Don't Get Bent Out of Shape

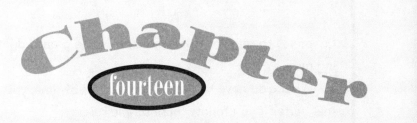

Chapter
fourteen

Sit on It

The long day on your duff begins the minute you sit up in bed. Then you sit on the john, at the dining table, in your car, at your desk, in meetings, and finally on the couch. You probably don't mind sitting down all day because it's pretty effortless to do. The problem lies (or should I say sits) in that even though sitting is easy, it's hard on your body.

Sitting puts a lot of stress on your back and hinders your posture and circulation. That's why you need to shape up the way you sit. It doesn't take much; taking a few precautions and moving a little will do the trick. So get ready to combat the wear and tear from too much time spent on your derriere!

THIRTY MINUTES ON YOUR DUFF IS QUITE ENOUGH

Sitting (especially in a static position) puts a huge load on the back. That's why you don't want to spend much more than 30 minutes on your seat without getting up and moving around. Sometimes getting up and moving is a little impossible (like when you're in the center of the row at the movies!). If you can't get up, be sure to do a lot of fidgeting. Just turn to

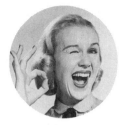

Chapter 9 to refresh your memory of some great fidgeting moves.

When you have to sit for long periods of time, you'll feel better if you follow these simple rules:

- Never settle into one position. Vary your seated positions every 15 minutes or so to lessen the stress on your back and maintain your posture.

- Set a timer on your watch or computer to remind you to get off your seat. You don't have to wander away from your desk every time. Just stand up and stretch, if you'd like.

- Move your file cabinet across the room so you have to walk over to it. You might as well do the same thing for your printer, stapler, and pencil sharpener.

- Stroll over to your co-worker's desk and give them the message instead of sending an E-mail.

- Place a rolled towel under the back edge of your buttocks to restore the natural curve in your spine. This strategy really helps when you have to drive for a long time.

- Speaking of driving, make sure you take pit stops during long trips. Plan to get out of the car and move around every hour. You can always drink lots of water so that you have to make a pit stop!

- Stand up when you're on the subway. (That's why the poles are there.)

- Check your posture regularly. At least once or twice an hour, incorporate any of the posture moves described later in this chapter.

LET'S GET COMFY

If you have to sit for a long time, you may as well get comfy. Most chairs can create excessive stress on your spine and the muscles of your legs, back, and neck. For the best comfort and support, your chair should fit the contours of your body. How you hold your body can make a big difference too. Here are some tips to keep you comfy from the top of your head to the bottom of your feet:

- **Your head and neck:** You should be able to look straight ahead at your computer screen. When you read, bring whatever you're reading up to your field of vision. When you talk on the phone, bring the handset up to your ear and mouth; don't bend your head and neck down or cradle the handset between your ear and neck.

- **Your spine:** Don't slouch! Sit up as straight as possible, keeping your buttocks and upper legs centered on the seat. Your upper body should rest against the seat back. If possible, get a chair with lumbar support to restore the natural curve of your spine and minimize pressure on your disks.

- **Your arms:** Make sure your chair has armrests. They can relieve pressure on your lower back and pulls on your neck and shoulders. Keep your arms parallel to the floor when using a keyboard and support them with the armrest as much as possible.

- **Your buttocks:** You want to sit squarely, which means you should avoid sitting on your wallet, car

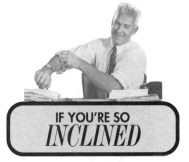

IF YOU'RE SO INCLINED

The next time you pull into a rest stop during a long drive you can relieve your muscles and joints and get the blood flowing by doing step-ups on the curb or a bench.

keys, checkbook, or anything else you have in your back pockets (tissue is okay). Sitting squarely will keep you from tipping your pelvis.

- **Your legs:** Don't cross your legs! If you must, do it at the ankles only. When your work requires reading, writing, or using the phone or calculator, lean forward so that your knees drop lower than your hips. (Tilt your chair forward 15 degrees if it's adjustable.) Be sure to keep your abdominals pulled in.

- **Your feet:** Whenever possible, keep your feet flat on the floor. Take off your high heels when you are at your desk. If you'd like, elevate your feet (one at a time) on a chair rung or small stool in front of you.

STAND UP FOR YOURSELF

Because I'm telling you not to sit so much, you'll probably be standing more. That's great! But just as you need to support your body when you sit, you must do the same while you stand. Use these tips to stand at ease:

- Keep your body relaxed and in your neutral position; your back should not be too flat (hips slouched forward) or too arched (hips tilted way back), but somewhere in the middle, with your buttocks tucked in slightly.

- Always keep your abdominals pulled in.

- Let your neck lengthen and become vertical; keep your head over your shoulders, with your chin slightly in.

- Never lock your knees. Always keep a slight bend in them.
- Vary your stance often. You can shift your weight from foot to foot as long as you keep your pelvis level.
- Lose the high heels. They put too much weight on the front of the foot, which in turn puts too much stress on your back.

POSE FOR YOUR POSTURE

When you don't think about your posture, you usually end up with rounded shoulders, a caved-in chest, a stiff neck, and a protruding stomach by the end of the day. If you don't think about it at all, you can start the day that way. Please take the time to find just the right pose for your posture. The following moves will point you in the right direction:

Moves to Improve Your Seat Time

Your head, neck, and back can get the most out of whack when you log in too much time on your seat. Do the following exercises, and you'll improve your chances of staying in one piece:

- Find your neutral position. This position is where your body is the most stable and comfortable. Stand or sit with your legs slightly apart and slowly rotate your pelvis forward as far as it will go. Now bring it back to center and tilt it as far backwards as it will go, and then bring it back to center. Shifting your

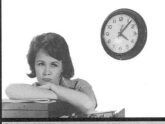

A COMPLETE WASTE OF TIME

The 3 Worst Ways to Stand (other than "corrected"):

1. With locked knees.
2. In high heels.
3. On your head.

Cut the cord! Save yourself from a stiff neck by using the speaker phone or a headset when talking on the phone. That way, you can also spend your time moving around instead of staying connected to a cord.

pelvis to the extremes makes you aware of what feels more stable, comfortable, and neutral.

- Nod your head. Place the palms of your hands on your head just behind and above your ears. Gently extend your neck upward as if a string is pulling you from the top of your skull. Then begin nodding your head, moving your forehead forward and your chin toward your chest.

- Fortify your neck. The best way to do this is to add some resistance without moving your head and neck. Clasp your hands behind your head and gently push backward with your head as you simultaneously push against it with equal pressure from your hands. Don't push too hard. You can do the same thing by pushing your hands against your forehead and pushing your head against your hands.

- Strengthen your lower back. A sure way to help your posture is to keep your lower back strong. Incorporate effective back strengthening exercises such as lower back arches (Chapter 10, p. 110), lying down arches (Chapter 10, p. 109), trunk raises (Chapter 12, p. 151), spinal stabilizers (Chapter 15, p. 180), and pull-ins (Chapter 13, p. 160) into your strength training.

Moves to Relieve Your Seat Time

Relieving your body from the stress of sitting will energize your muscles, improve your circulation, and rejuvenate you all over. The great thing is you don't even have to leave your chair. You can do the following stretches right at your desk:

- Roll your shoulders. Move your shoulders backwards in a large circular pattern. Do this as smoothly as possible. You can also move one shoulder at a time.

- Reach up. Stretch your arms upward and slightly behind you. Take a deep breath and exhale. Circle your wrists in both directions a few times and then bring your arms back down.

- Press your shoulders down. Gently press your shoulders down as if someone were standing on top of them. Hold for a count of five and then release. Do this exercise a couple of times.

- Bend your back. Place your palms on your lower back and lean backward. Hold for a count of five and then straighten back up. Repeat this exercise a few times. It's a great stretch to do while you're standing, too.

- Roll forward. This stretch helps relax your lower back. Be sure to have your knees and feet apart (feet flat on floor) and keep your back straight for this move. Slowly bend forward as far as you comfortably can. Hold this position for a count of 10, and then slowly return to an upright position.

Chapter 16 describes lots of other stretches you can do to relieve the stress on your body that comes from sitting.

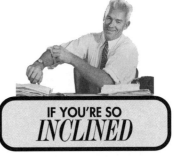

IF YOU'RE SO
INCLINED

Go stand in the corner! If you want to ease the stiffness in your upper back and shoulders, just go and face the corner of a room. Stretch your arms back with palms holding on to the walls as you let your body lean forward.

Getting Time on Your Side

	The Old Way	The Lazy Way
Sitting still in your seat	For hours	No more than 30 minutes
Finding a comfortable sitting position	Never really do	Seconds
Finding a comfortable standing position	Never really do	Seconds
Getting rid of a stiff neck	All day	A few minutes
Getting rid of a stiff back	All day	A few minutes
Relieving back pain	Days (and lots of pills)	A few minutes

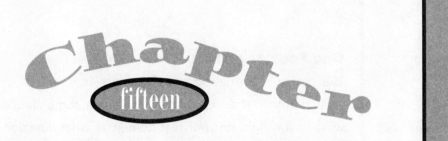

The Perfect Balance

Balance is an elusive state of being. How can you be balanced when you're constantly being pulled in all directions? Suppose you are being pulled, literally. Do you think you can stand your ground or will you topple over?

Being able to stay balanced (physically, although it wouldn't hurt to be emotionally balanced as well) is a big part of being in shape. It's what keeps you centered as you do any activity. When you can maintain your balance, you enhance your performance, improve your reaction time, and prevent injuries. It doesn't take much to stay balanced (again, I'm talking physically, not emotionally). You just mix a little imagination with some exercises and do what comes naturally.

DON'T BE LEFT WITH TWO LEFT FEET

I know what you're thinking—perfect balance is only for ballerinas, gymnasts, yogis, and ice skaters, right? Wrong! Balance is not a special talent shared by a few. It can be learned. You just need to concentrate a little and challenge your balance as often as you can.

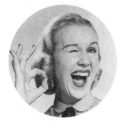

QUICK ◧ PAINLESS

One Foot at a Time

The best way to develop your balance is to test it in motion rather than in stillness. Here are some simple ways to stay light on your feet no matter what direction you're going:

- A game of Twister or hopscotch
- Martial arts (for example, Tai Chi, yoga, or Judo)
- Jumping rope one-legged
- Balance beam exercises
- Minitrampolining (the big one's more fun, but less safe)
- Walking on stilts
- Lunging, hopping, springing, leaping
- Aerobic dancing
- Ballet
- Gymnastics
- Kickboxing
- A game of "Red Light, Green Light" (you have to stop on one leg though)
- Any of the balancing exercises in this book

Take It One Step Further

Balance starts every time you move out of that center position; in doing so, you challenge your body to stabilize itself. There are lots of ways you can test your balancing ability, but these are some of the most effective ones:

- Close your eyes
- Use one leg only
- Don't use arms
- Vary your surface (for example, use sand or a ball)
- Increase your range of motion
- Increase your speed

DO WHAT COMES NATURALLY

When choosing an aerobic activity, you can get more out of your efforts if you do what comes naturally. Walking, running, or riding outdoors will give you a key benefit that their machine counterparts (treadmill, stationary bike) do not offer. When you do these activities naturally, you force your body to balance and stabilize itself instead of relying on a machine to stabilize you.

By taking it outdoors, you not only improve your coordination and balance, you also enhance the pleasure of your workout. You are much more apt to keep at it in nature than in a confined space. Heck, you might even go a little longer.

There's nothing wrong with climbing on a machine for your workout. Going to a gym or recreation center can give you structure, camaraderie, variety, and a dry place in bad weather. But if you want to improve your balance and coordination, do what comes naturally.

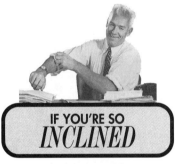

IF YOU'RE SO
INCLINED

Fashion yourself as a flamingo. Challenge your balance by doing daily tasks such as brushing your teeth or washing the dishes on one leg. You might not want to stand too far away from the counter!

BALANCING ACTS

The exercises in this section will develop your balance. I threw the ball in again because a stability ball is one of the best tools for challenging your equilibrium. So give yourself a dare and see how long you can stand with one leg in the air.

The Spinal Stabilizer

This exercise strengthens the muscles that support the lower (lumbar) part of your spine. It's an excellent one to do to balance your body and keep your spine straight.

1. Get down on all fours, with your hands directly under your shoulders and your knees under your hips. Look down, keeping your head aligned with your spine and your back straight (no arch).

2. Lift and extend your right arm and left leg, keeping both parallel to the floor. Hips should stay level. Count to 10.

3. Slowly lower your right arm and left leg, and then lift and extend your left arm and right leg.

4. Repeat each side 8 to 10 times.

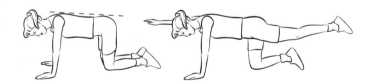

Spinal stabilizer.

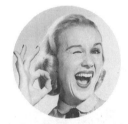

QUICK ☺ PAINLESS

The spinal stabilizer is one exercise you shouldn't try to do without. Between heavy bags, sitting all day, and general stress, we wreak havoc on our backs. This exercise only takes a few minutes so do it for you and your back!

Flamingos

Doing this exercise may not make you as perfectly poised as a flamingo, but it definitely will improve your balance.

1. Stand up straight, with your body relaxed and arms to your side. Lift your right leg up behind you with your heel pointing toward your buttocks. Keep your hips level. All of your weight is now on your left leg. Hold this position for a count of 20 to 30.

2. Bring your right leg down and switch sides, putting all of your weight on the right leg. Be sure to keep your body straight (shoulders over hips).

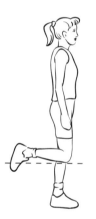

Flamingos.

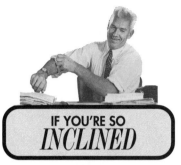

IF YOU'RE SO
INCLINED

Ready for more of a challenge? Try adding some ankle weights into this exercise and increase your resistance.

Sit and March on a Ball

It's hard to march when you are sitting down, let alone sitting on an unstable surface, such as an exercise ball. This exercise will help strengthen your leg muscles as it challenges your balance.

1. Sit on the ball in a neutral position (back is neither too arched nor too flat).

2. Begin marching in a rhythmic manner, swinging your opposite arm with your opposite leg.

3. Continue this movement until you get tired or lose form.

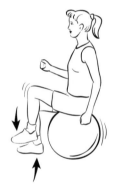

Sitting and marching on a ball.

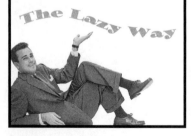

Congratulations! You didn't fall off when you marched on the ball. Now march on down to the nearest Baskin-Robbins and get yourself a low-fat treat.

The Lazy Way

Balance on Ball with No Hands or Feet

Remember when you used to take your hands off the handlebars when riding your bike? This balancing exercise should bring it all back to you.

1. Sit on the ball in a neutral position.

2. Extend your arms straight out to the sides of your body (keep a slight bend in your elbows).

3. Slowly lift and extend your legs away from the ball. Be careful not to overextend them. Hold the position for as long as you can.

4. Yell, "Look, Ma, no hands or feet!"

Make sure you do this in a clear area (no table corners in reach) when you try it for the first time—balance takes practice, but we'd like to make sure it doesn't involve any bruises when you try!

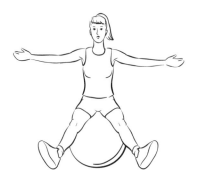

Balancing on a ball with no hands or feet.

Balance Ball on Feet

This exercise will get you ready for the circus! You'll get a kick out of how challenging balancing a ball can be.

1. Lie on your back.

2. Bend your knees toward your chest, making your lower legs perpendicular to your torso.

3. Place the ball on the soles of your feet and then bring your arms down by your sides.

4. Straighten your knees and raise the ball toward the ceiling, keeping it balanced on your feet.

5. Lower your knees back to your chest and repeat the exercise 5 to 10 times.

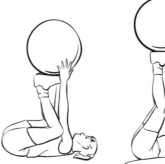
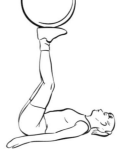

Balancing a ball on the feet.

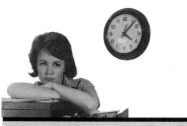

A COMPLETE WASTE OF TIME

The 3 Worst Places to Try Out Your New Balancing Act:

1. In the middle of the road.

2. At the top of the stairs.

3. On a ladder.

THIS YOGI SALUTE WILL TURN YOU INTO ONE COORDINATED BEAUT

Most martial arts disciplines require coordination and balance, not just for the actual movements, but also to harmonize body, mind, and breathing. This type of activity enhances your agility as well as your concentration (and hopefully, karma). That's why I'm giving you a yoga exercise routine (sun salutation) that's been around since the first yogi. It will definitely challenge your coordination, but it will leave you feeling refreshed. Don't worry, you won't have to turn into a pretzel with this routine.

1. Stand up straight and relaxed. Bring the palms of your hands together in front of your chest (the heart center) as if you were praying. Inhale and exhale slowly and smoothly.

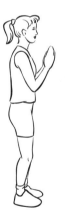

Position one.

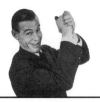

Go natural in Mother Nature! Choose to bike outside instead of using the stationary cycle. That way, you'll force your body to balance and stabilize itself.

2. Cross your thumbs and raise your arms straight out in front of you, then bring them up over your head. Inhale as you look up and bend slightly backward. Do a pelvic tilt when you lift your arms over your head in order to protect your back.

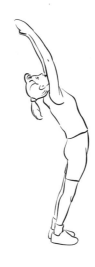

Position two.

3. Exhale as you bend forward from the hips, keeping your back straight. You can bend your knees a little if you need to.

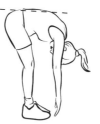

Position three.

4. Bring the palms of your hands flat on the floor (go ahead and bend your knees to accomplish this), and then stretch one leg straight back behind you, allowing the knee to rest on the floor. The other knee is bent with the lower part of it perpendicular to the floor. Look up and inhale.

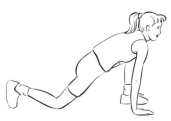

Position four.

5. Move the front leg backward to meet the other, your weight resting on your hands and feet. You can keep your hips high (body looks like an upside-down V) or low (body is parallel to floor).

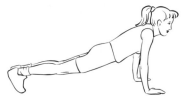

Position five.

6. Lower your knees, chest, and chin to the floor. Keep your hips raised even though the rest of your body parts are flat on the floor. Exhale completely.

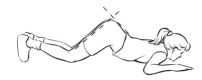

Position six.

7. Pressing on the palms of your hands, push your body back up to position five. Keep hips high and distribute weight on your palms and feet (flat).

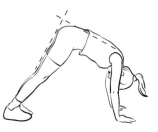

Position seven.

8. Step one leg forward, bringing your foot between both hands. Drop the knee of the other leg and lift your chest while looking upward. Inhale.

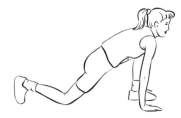

Position eight.

9. Move your back foot forward, next to the other one. You should now be back in position three. Exhale.

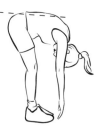

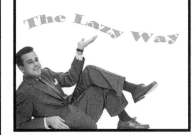
Position nine.

10. Lift your hands off the floor into the proper position with thumbs locked. Extend your arms straight out and up, leading your body into a standing position. Arms are now above your head alongside your ears.

Position ten.

11. Repeat position two, inhaling as you look up and bend slightly backward.

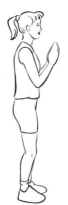

Position eleven.

12. Finish the salutation by bringing your arms down in front of the chest, keeping your palms together. Exhale and inhale slowly and smoothly.

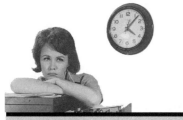

Position twelve.

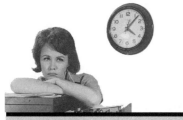

A COMPLETE WASTE OF TIME

The 3 Worst Things to Do on One Leg:

1. Walk the trapeze.

2. Ride a unicycle.

3. Kick someone.

You can do several repetitions of this exercise. It is an excellent way to warm up your muscles before your aerobic or strength activities. There are many variations of this salutation; for instance, you can do it slowly, or you can jump rapidly from one pose to the other. My recommendation is for you to do it *The Lazy Way,* which is slow and easy.

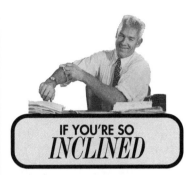

IF YOU'RE SO
INCLINED

Do this salutation first thing in the morning to slowly wake up your body, muscle by muscle. You'll feel energized and ready to face the day!

Getting Time on Your Side

	The Old Way	The Lazy Way
Balancing on one leg	Lots of wasted time trying	2 minutes or more
Balancing on one arm and one leg	Lots of wasted time trying	2 minutes or more
Doing your balancing exercises	20 minutes	5 minutes
Doing your sun salutation	20 minutes (because you had to keep starting over)	5 minutes
Balancing on machines	All the time	No time
Balancing your exercise routine	Lots of wasted time trying	30 minutes

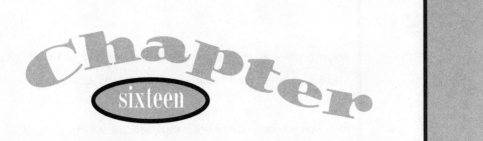

Unleashers and Releasers

It seems you're always stretched for time when it comes to getting in your flexibility exercises. It's not like you don't do any stretches. You put on your socks and reach for the remote control quite regularly. But if you could just add a few more stretches in your day, your body would greatly appreciate it.

Stretching keeps you limber and helps prevent back, neck, and shoulder pain. When you don't regularly stretch, your muscles and connective tissues tend to lose their elastic ability. After a sedentary day in front of the computer, you probably know exactly what that loss feels like. So how about a few stretches to stave off the stiffness and help you unwind?

DON'T OVERSTRETCH YOUR BOUNDARIES

Stretching can improve your flexibility and prevent you from getting injured, but you need to do it the right way. If you don't, you can do your body more harm than good. Use these guidelines to avoid overstretching your boundaries:

- Stretch only after your muscles are warmed up. It's even better if you stretch after you exercise because your muscles are most warm and loose then.

- Always stretch slowly and gradually (never forcefully) up to a point of tension (a slight stretching or pulling sensation). This should feel like your muscles are pulling just a bit beyond what they're used to.

- Never stretch beyond the tension point to where you feel pain.

- Use proper form and concentrate on the muscle being stretched.

- Hold each stretch for 30 to 60 counts.

- Never bounce!

- Stretch regularly, at least three times a week.

MOVES TO RELEASE YOUR UPPER BODY

Are you tired of feeling like the hunchback of Notre Dame? You don't have to be a prisoner to tight upper body muscles if you let the following moves release you.

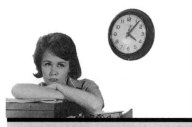

A COMPLETE WASTE OF TIME

The 3 Worst Things to Do to Your Muscles When You Stretch:

1. Bounce them.

2. Keep them cold (always warm them up first).

3. Overstretch them.

Neck Unleashers

This stretch is for your neck and boy does it feel good after a long day in front of the computer.

1. Stand erect, with your arms dangling at your sides.

2. Tilt your head to your right side. Lower your right ear to your right shoulder while keeping your shoulders down. Hold this position.

3. Repeat this movement to the left side.

4. Turn your head to the right with your chin pointing toward your shoulders (shoulders remain still). Hold this position.

5. Repeat this movement to the left side.

6. Pull in your chin to make a "double" chin, stretching the back of your neck. Hold this position. **Caution:** Do not lift your chin up and tilt your head back while doing this, or you will hyperextend your neck.

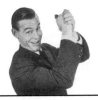

If a little is good, then more must be better, right? Not so when it comes to stretching. Do yourself a favor and don't overstretch your muscles. They'll thank you for it later.

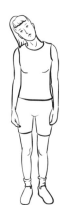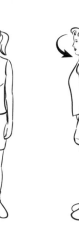

Neck unleashers.

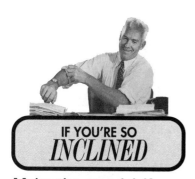

Make the rounds! If you like circling your shoulders for a stretch, then you'll love doing arm circles for an exercise. Just hold your arms straight out from your side and begin moving them in circles. Start with small ones and make them bigger as you go.

Shoulder Slackeners

This stretch will help loosen up your shoulders, especially when they're tight from prolonged periods of sitting.

1. Move your shoulders in a circle. Start with five forward circles, and then do five backward circles.

2. Stretch your right arm across your chest with your left hand pressing against your right arm. Hold this position.

3. Repeat the movement with your left arm.

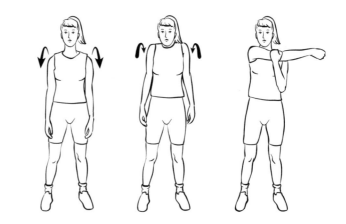

Shoulder slackeners.

Upper Back Unbinders

You won't want to stop doing this stretch once you get the hang of it.

1. While you bend your elbows, interlock your fingers in front of your chest, with your palms outward.

2. Push your arms forward, straightening your arms and rounding your upper back. Hold this position, and then release it.

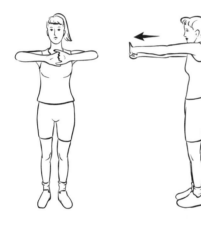

Upper back unbinders.

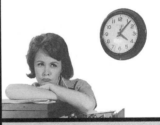

A COMPLETE WASTE OF TIME

The 3 Worst Things to Stretch:

1. Your patience.
2. Your tolerance.
3. Your cat.

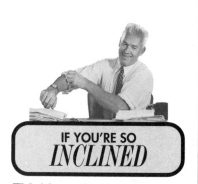

Chest Openers

This move will give you a nice stretch in your chest and the front of your shoulders.

1. Stand next to a wall, positioning your body parallel to the wall and a little less than an arm's length away from it. Start with left side being closest to the wall.

2. Place your left hand on the wall at shoulder height. Your arm should be extended with a slight bend at your elbow.

3. Keeping your left hand and both feet in place, begin turning your torso away from the wall until you feel a gentle stretch in your chest.

4. Repeat this exercise with your right side closest to the wall.

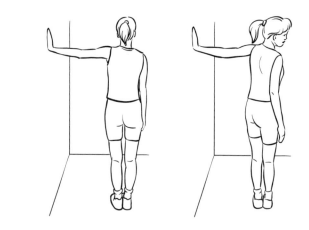

Chest openers.

Arm Relaxers

This stretch targets the back of your arms.

1. With your left hand, pull your right elbow behind your head. Your right elbow will be sticking up behind your head.

2. With your left hand gently pushing down on your right elbow, stretch the fingers of your right hand down your back. Hold this position.

3. Do the same stretch on the other side.

4. For a deeper stretch, grasp a towel with your right hand and bend your right elbow, dangling the towel down the center of your back.

5. Place your left hand behind your back and reach up to grab the towel end.

6. Gradually move your hands closer together. Hold this position.

7. Do the same stretch on the other side.

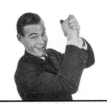

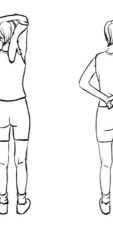

Arm relaxers.

YOU'LL THANK YOURSELF LATER

If your arms are beginning to feel as though they're going to drop off from exercising, give them a feel-good stretch by doing arm relaxers. While you're at it, give yourself a hug, too.

MOVES TO UNLEASH YOUR LOWER BODY

A day of sitting can tighten up the legs and lower back. Your best defense (besides having good posture) is to get on the floor and do the following stretches. They'll unleash your lower body in no time.

Knee Huggers

This stretch is great for the times you want to just curl up in a ball and lie down.

1. Lie on your back with your knees bent, your feet flat on the floor, and your arms straight out to the sides.

2. Bring your knees toward your chest and keep them bent at a right angle; hug them with your arms. Hold this position.

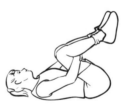

Knee huggers.

Plop-Overs

You'll feel this stretch down the side of your back and into your hips. Be sure to go slowly and stay controlled.

1. Start with the knee huggers, but leave your arms straight out to the sides.

2. Keeping both shoulders on the floor, slowly let your legs fall to the right side until your right leg is resting on the floor. Hold this position.

3. Repeat this stretch on the other side.

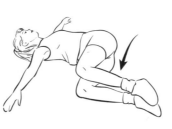

Plop-overs.

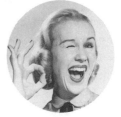

QUICK ⚫ PAINLESS

No time to lie down? You don't have to get on your back to stretch your hamstrings. You can also stretch them standing up. Just place one leg in front of you with heel down and toes up. Bend forward from the hips, hold the stretch, and then switch legs.

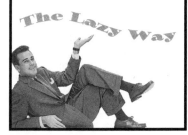
Back Leg Looseners

Back leg looseners are great stretches to do after a brisk walk or run. They are also important to do after a day of sitting because tight hamstrings can pull on the lower back.

1. Lying on your back, slowly raise your right leg, clasping your hands under your right thigh. Your left leg is straight with your left heel resting on the floor.

2. Gently pull your right leg toward your chest, keeping it straight. Hold this position.

3. Repeat the stretch with your left leg.

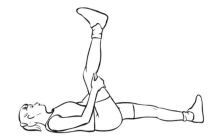

Back leg looseners.

Front Leg Looseners

This stretch is your best bet for loosening the muscles at the front of your thigh.

1. Lie on your left side with your legs straight and your left knee bent slightly forward.

2. Grasp your right foot or ankle with your right hand and gently pull your right leg backward without arching your back.

3. If you are not troubled by knee problems, pull your right heel gently toward your buttocks during this stretch. Hold this position.

4. Repeat the stretch for the other side.

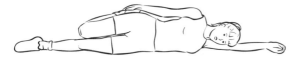

Front leg looseners.

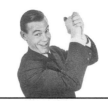

YOU'LL THANK YOURSELF LATER

No matter what, stretch both before and after exercising—your muscles will be grateful, and you'll avoid injuries!

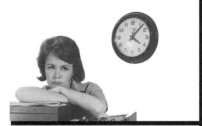

Hip Unflexors

This stretch targets the muscles that are contracted the whole time you are sitting. It's a must if your day is sedentary.

1. Get down on your left knee as if you were going to propose marriage. Your right knee should be at a right angle to the floor, with the knee over the ankle.

2. Without moving your right leg, press your hips forward until you feel a stretch in the upper part of your left thigh. Don't let your back arch.

3. Repeat the stretch with the other leg.

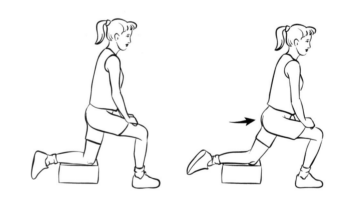

Hip unflexors.

Ease Into Its

This move will give you a great stretch in the back of your lower legs. Your calves will especially love this stretch after you go for a run.

1. Stand erect, with your arms dangling at your sides.

2. Step forward on your left foot, with your right leg resting on toes pointed straight forward.

3. Press your right heel to the floor, keeping your left knee aligned over your left ankle. To deepen the stretch, slide your right foot farther backward. Hold this position.

4. Now, slightly bend your back knee without lifting your heel. Hold this position.

5. Repeat the same process for the other side.

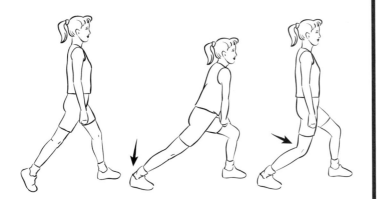

Ease into its.

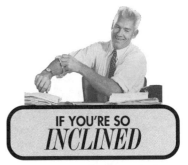

IF YOU'RE SO INCLINED

If you spend a lot of time standing during the day, do this stretch every hour or so. You'll find your legs and feet will be less sore by the time you get home.

MOVES TO UNLOCK YOUR BACK

This section describes even more stretches to squeeze the tension out of your back. The difference between these and the ones described in Chapter 14 (moves to relieve your seat time) is that you have to get down on the floor. This might put you on the spot if you did them at the office.

Up and Down Arches

Some people call this the cat stretch, and that's fine by me because cats sure know what they're doing when it comes to stretching.

1. Get down on your hands and knees.

2. Arch your back up like a scared cat. Pull your stomach in and hold this position.

3. Lower your back until it bows in the middle. Hold this position.

4. Repeat this stretch as many times as you like.

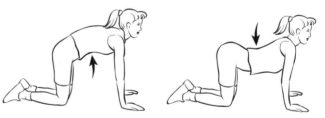

Up and down arches.

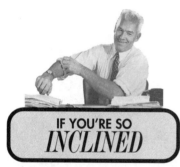

Back Releasers

This stretch will help ease the stiffness in your lower back:

1. Lie on your stomach with your palms on the floor slightly forward of your shoulders.

2. Relax your back and slowly press up your body for a good back and abdominal stretch.

3. Keep hips on floor and eyes looking straight ahead (not up). Hold this position.

4. Lower yourself back down to the floor. If you start to feel pain in your lower back, either do not lift as high or discontinue the stretch.

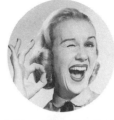

QUICK 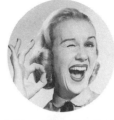 *PAINLESS*

Stretch those knots right out! Try this during your lunch break and you'll feel rejuvenated for the rest of the day!

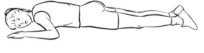

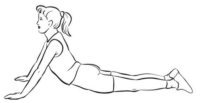

Back releasers.

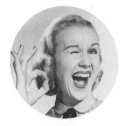

Lying Down Liberators

It's hard not to yawn when you do this stretch, which is, incidentally, a great move to do while you're sitting or standing, too.

1. Lie down with your back on the floor, extending your arms over your head.

2. Point your toes and give your body a full stretch as if you are being pulled from both ends.

3. Hold stretch and then relax.

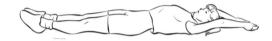

Lying down liberators.

Getting Time on Your Side

	The Old Way	The Lazy Way
Stretching your neck	2 minutes	30 to 60 seconds
Stretching your shoulders	3 minutes	30 to 60 seconds
Stretching your chest	2 minutes	30 to 60 seconds
Stretching your back	10 minutes	5 minutes
Stretching your arms	5 minutes	30 to 60 seconds
Stretching your legs	10 minutes	5 minutes

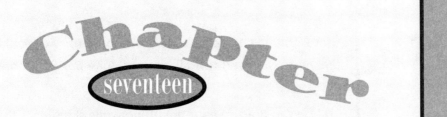
Now It's Time to Relax

Our bodies are probably the most perfectly designed machines on earth, but they are not ever-ready bunnies that can keep going and going—thank God! How could we relax if we were wound up all the time? We just have to call it quits every now and then and give ourselves some rest and relaxation.

Rest and relaxation are vital for keeping you from getting overworked, sick, or insane. Instead, they'll put a spring in your step and a smile on your face. Forget about everything else, because now it's time to relax! In this chapter, you'll learn how to breathe deeply, de-stress your life, and keep your energy level up all day long. You'll also discover the importance of the mind-body-spirit connection and the many pay-offs of shaping up.

TAKE A DEEP BREATH

Breathing is one of those things we don't give much thought to. We know we're doing it, so we tend to turn our focus elsewhere. What most of us don't realize is that if we

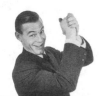

Listen to your body! If you're having to drag it around with you as you go at warp speed, it won't be doing you any favors. But you're not doing it any favors either. The next time your body starts to drag, slow down and get some rest and relaxation.

concentrated on taking some deep breaths, we would feel more calm and revitalized and, quite possibly, more alive!

1. You can practice your breathing while standing, sitting, or lying down. The main thing is to keep your body relaxed. Try it with your eyes closed.

2. Place the palm of one hand on your abdomen and your other palm on your chest. This will help you be more aware of your breathing pattern.

3. Slowly inhale through the nose, focusing attention on your breath without trying to influence it.

4. As your abdomen expands slightly, feel your lower ribs move out to the sides. You should feel your diaphragm contract downward, which is what expands your lower abdomen. Your lower back should stay flat.

5. As you complete the breath in, notice how your upper chest expands as your lungs fill with air.

6. Exhale slowly through the mouth, feeling the air being squeezed out of your lungs and a wave of relaxation flowing through your abdomen, chest, throat, and face. The deeper you exhale, the more air you will breathe in.

7. Continue this breathing pattern, feeling the touch of air in your nose and the gentle, even in-and-out flow of inhalation and exhalation.

HAVE YOU HAD A BREAK TODAY?

A little stress now and then isn't necessarily a bad thing. In fact, it can rev you up to meet any challenge. Stress only becomes a problem when you can't manage it or you keep it bottled up inside. So how can you deal with stress? Just give yourself a break! Try these few simple ways to defuse the stress in your life:

- Switch from A to B. No sense in being the impatient, workaholic type, especially when it may increase your risk for heart disease. Learn to be a little more mellow and live for the moment.

- Drop a few things. Don't feel pressured to do too many things at once or spread yourself too thin. Just say no! Or delegate certain tasks to others.

- Give yourself a time-out. Find a quiet comfortable place with no distractions and stay there for a few minutes. You can practice your breathing, meditate, or pray. Or you might prefer a more active time-out activity, such as pummeling a punching bag (hey, whatever works).

- Get a massage. There's nothing like a good rubdown to melt away the tension. It can release a tight back or neck and even get rid of headaches.

- Take a vacation in your mind. When there's no place you can go to get away from it all, take a trip inside your head. Through the power of visualization and imagination, you can visit your favorite places without it costing you a penny!

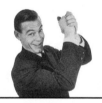

YOU'LL THANK YOURSELF LATER

Take a load off! If you feel yourself beginning to cave in under the pressure, do yourself a favor and lighten your load. Delegate tasks to others and then go get a massage.

Give yourself a wave of relaxation. You can relieve tense spots in your body by doing progressive muscle relaxation. Start at your toes and work your way up the body, tensing each muscle for about five seconds and then releasing and relaxing it for 10 to 15 seconds.

Smile! Even the slightest smile will increase blood flow to the brain and reverse negative thoughts. Laughing will increase this effect a hundredfold.

Don't forget to exercise! Doing something physical is an excellent way to dissipate stress. It also helps strengthen the body's ability to meet stressful demands. Exercise also releases those wonderful endorphins.

RECHARGE YOURSELF ALL DAY LONG

Sometimes it just takes a splash of ice water on your face (other times, it may take a whole ice bath) to recharge yourself. That seems to work, at least until the next lull rolls around. Take a look at these guidelines to help prevent your energy from going down the drain.

Eat early and often. If you want to keep fuel in your engine, you need to eat small, wholesome meals throughout the day, starting with breakfast. Remember that it's better to eat during the active hours of your day rather than when your body's winding down or sleeping.

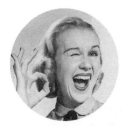

QUICK PAINLESS

Make your own happy drugs! Just a few minutes of vigorous exercise is all it takes to produce endorphins, which will make you feel euphoric.

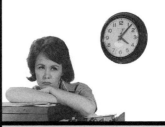

- Drink lots of water! Becoming dehydrated is very fatiguing on the body. Getting enough water helps your body run cool.

- Go easy on the caffeine. Too much of this stimulant can leave you in a state of fatigue or nervous irritability. The same thing goes for ginseng, ephedrine, and phenylpropanolamine (stimulant in appetite suppressants).

- Lay off the sugar. Too much refined sugar or flour during the day will peak your energy for a bit, but then it'll come crashing down. Stick to real, wholesome foods, and if you need something sweet, have a piece of fruit.

- Get a good night's sleep. When you don't get enough sleep, you hinder your concentration and performance. If you can't get in a full night's rest, try taking a power nap during the day!

- Don't get comfortable. Remember, if you have to sit a lot, get up and move around frequently and always fidget when you get the chance.

- Change the scenery. You can recharge yourself by taking a few moments to get away from whatever you're doing. Go get a drink of water, visit with a co-worker, or just stop outside for a breath of fresh air.

- Stretch your body. Choose from any of the flexibility exercises described in this book or do the "sun salutation" described in Chapter 15. You'll feel revived and ready to keep on going and going.

A COMPLETE WASTE OF TIME

The 3 Worst Ways to Recharge Yourself:

1. Sticking your finger in a light socket.

2. Drinking a triple shot of espresso.

3. Babysitting 10 little boys.

IT'S AN EASY FLIP OF THE SWITCH FOR YOUR MIND-BODY-SPIRIT CONNECTION

Sure, shaping up can tone your muscles and help you get into your jeans. But, more importantly, the process of getting in shape can make your mind, body, and spirit work in harmony. Here are a few tips to help you get connected:

▨ Set realistic but challenging goals. When you get out of your comfort zone, you discover a deeper layer of yourself. Setting and achieving your goals is one of the best ways to boost your self-confidence and let your spirit soar.

▨ Tune in to your natural rhythm. Be conscious of your breathing and movements. The more you do, the more natural it will be for you to get into "automatic mode" as you work out. This mode is your mind, body, and spirit working in perfect harmony.

▨ Learn how to meditate. Meditation calms your body, focuses your mind, and fills you with a peaceful alertness. The key is to quiet your mind and empty it of all thoughts. Think you can do that?

▨ Motivate yourself. Read an inspirational story. Train for an athletic event. Fill your mind with positive thoughts. These thoughts will motivate you to be all that you can be.

▨ Don't get hung up on your weight. Focus on getting fit, and the weight loss will be a fringe benefit. It's important that you learn to love your body no matter what size or shape it is. Remember, it's the inside (spirit) that counts.

- Get out into nature. Nature is the queen of playgrounds. It's the perfect place to keep you in touch with your spirit. It's awesome; it's tranquil; it's healthy!

- Renew yourself each day. Take a few moments each day to remind yourself that you are alive. Reflect on your goals and what you are going to do to accomplish them. Renewing your mind, body, and spirit on a daily basis will help you shape up your life.

THE PAYOFFS OF SHAPING UP

Shaping up (even *The Lazy Way*) is more about health than beauty. That's because it enables you to work, play, and live. (You won't look too bad in a bikini either.) There's just no getting around it—shaping up is necessary if you want to feel good! Here are 20 reasons why shaping up pays off:

- Fat loss and muscle gain, which translates into a smaller, shapelier shape

- More energy

- Improved posture, which leads to improved physical appearance

- Alleviation of chronic lower pack pain

- Lower blood pressure and cholesterol

- Improved sleep

- Decreased appetite

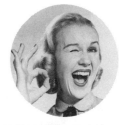

QUICK ☎ *PAINLESS*

Shape up or get old! If you want to slow down the aging process, get in some exercise. It might not add more years to your life, but it will definitely add more life to your years!

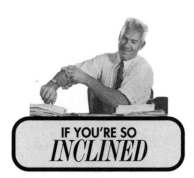

Don't hesitate to mediate! Take a few minutes each morning or evening to sit and quiet your mind. Just close your eyes and breathe deeply, focusing on your breath as it flows in and out. Don't let your attention wander from your breathing.

- Increased endurance and ability to withstand fatigue
- Elevated mood (even euphoric at times!)
- Boosted immune system
- Better circulation of blood and oxygen
- Improved digestion
- Healthier joints
- Better reaction time
- Stronger bones
- Increased flexibility, balance, and coordination
- Stabilized blood sugar
- Decreased stress
- Increased self-confidence
- Higher quality of life

Shaping up *The Lazy Way* will make you feel good, inside and out!

Getting Time on Your Side

	The Old Way	The Lazy Way
Taking a deep breath	Takes several breaths (and minutes)	One breath
Getting rid of stress	Never	Just a few minutes
Recharging your mind	All of your vacation time	Just a few minutes
Recharging your body	All of your vacation time	Just a few minutes
Recharging your spirit	All of your vacation time	Just a few minutes
Recharging your energy	All of your vacation time	Just a few minutes

More Lazy Stuff

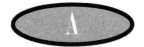

How to Get Someone Else to Do It

SHAPING UP YOUR EXERCISE PROGRAM

Whether you need a personal trainer, an aerobic instructor, various specialized programs or just a place to work out, these resources will help you shape up your exercise program.

- Aerobics & Fitness Association of America: (800) 365-5376
- American College of Sports Medicine: (317) 637-9200
- American Council on Exercise: (800) 529-8277
- American Running and Fitness Association: (800) 776-2732
- City recreation department
- Cooper Institute for Aerobic Research: (972) 701-8001
- International Spa and Fitness Association: (703) 838-2930
- Jazzercise: (800) 348-4748
- Local health clubs
- National Academy of Sports Medicine

- National Federation of Personal Trainers: (800) 729-6378

- National Strength and Conditioning Association: (719) 632-6722

- Women's Sports & Fitness Foundation: (212) 980-5580

- YMCA/YWCA

SHAPING UP YOUR DIET

The following organizations can help you organize your eating habits!

- American Diabetes Association (call local chapter for info)

- American Dietetic Association: (800) 366-1655 (This organization can give you a list of registered dieticians in your area.)

- American Heart Association: (800) 242-8721

- Center for Human Nutrition: (402) 559-5500

- Duke University Diet and Fitness Program: (800) 362-8446

- Hospitals (in-house weight-loss/eating programs)

- Johns Hopkins Weight Management Center: (410) 550-2330

- Stanford Weight Loss Risk and Reduction Program, Stanford University: (415) 723-5868

- Weight Control Center, New York Hospital: (212) 583-1000

- Weight Watchers International: (800) 651-6000

SHAPING UP YOUR HOME GYM

If you want to set up a home gym without any hassle, just do it *The Lazy Way* and use the resources below.

- Budget Cardio: (800) 929-4187

- Cybex: (800) 645-5392

- Dyna-Bands: (813) 951-0767

- Hydro-Fit Inc.: (541) 484-4361

- Fitness Wholesale Catalog: (888) 396-7337

- NordicTrack: (800) 468-4429

- Resist-A-Ball: (800) 476-8631

- Spri Performance Systems: (800) 488-7774

- StairMaster: (800) 635-2936

- Tectrix Fitness Equipment: (800) 767-8082

- Treadwall: (800) 707-9616

- Unisen, Inc.: (800) 228-6635

If You Really Want More, Read These

SHAPING UP YOUR EXERCISE PROGRAM

The following books, magazines and audios are great guides to get you moving, whatever way you choose.

ACSM. *ACSM Fitness Book.* Champaign, IL: Human Kinetics Pub., 1996.

Anderson, Bob. *Stretching.* Shelter Publications, 1987.

Bailey, Covert. *The Fit or Fat Woman.* Boston: Houghton Mifflin Co., 1989.

———. *The New Fit or Fat.* Boston: Houghton Mifflin Co., 1991.

———. *Smart Exercise.* Boston: Houghton Mifflin Co., 1996.

Bauer, Joy. *The Complete Idiot's Guide to Getting and Keeping Your Perfect Body.* New York: Macmillan Publishing.

Bicycling Magazine.

Birch, Beryl Bender. *Power Yoga: The Total Strength and Flexibility Workout.*

Bricklin, Mark. *Prevention's Practical Encyclopedia of Walking for Health: From Age-Reversal to Weight Loss, the Most Complete Guide Ever Written*. Emmans, PA: Rodale Press, 1993.

Burfoot, Amby. *Runner's World Complete Book of Running: Everything You Need to Know to Run for Fun, Fitness, and Competition*. Emmans, PA :Rodale Press, 1997.

Christensen, Alice. *The American Yoga Association Beginner's Manual*. Fireside, 1987.

Cooper, Kenneth H. *The Aerobics Program for Total Well-Being: Exercise, Diet, Emotional Balance*. New York: Bantam Doubleday Dell Pub., 1985.

Creager, Caroline Corning. *Therapeutic Exercises Using the Swiss Ball*. Boulder, CO: Executive Physical Therapy.

Edwards, Sally. *Sally Edwards' Heart Zone Training: Exercise Smart, Stay Fit, and Live Longer*. Adams Pub., 1996.

Fitzgerald, F. Stop. *The Fitness Log Book for Runners: The Essential Training Diary for Runners, Walkers, and Triathletes*. Thunder's Mouth Pr., 1997.

Fixx, James F. *The Complete Book of Running*. Random House, 1977.

Galloway, Jeff. *Galloway's Book on Running*. Bolinas, CA: Shelter Publications, Inc., 1984.

Greene, Bob. *A Journal of Daily Renewal: The Companion to Make the Connection*. New York: Hyperion Books, 1996.

———. *Make the Connection: Ten Steps to a Better Body and a Better Life*. New York: Hyperion Books, 1996.

Ho'o, Marshall. *Tai Chi Chuan*. Irvine, CA: Karl-Loriman Video, 1989.

Katz, Jane. *Swimming for Total Fitness*. New York: Doubleday Dolphin, 1993.

Kybartas, Ray. *Fitness Is Religion: Keep the Faith*. New York: Simon & Schuster, 1997.

Living Fit Magazine.

Martins, Peter. *The New York City Ballet Workout: Fifty Stretches and Exercises Anyone Can Do for a Strong, Graceful, and Sculpted Body*. William Morrow & Company, 1997.

Men's Fitness Magazine.

Mountain Bike Magazine.

Nelson, Miriam E. *Strong Women Stay Young*. New York: Bantam Books, 1997.

Pang, Chia Siew and Hock, Goh Ewe. *Tai Chi: Ten Minutes To Health*. CRCS Publications, 1988.

Penn State Sports Medicine Newsletter.

Peterson, James A. *Strength Training for Women*. Champaign, IL: Human Kinetics Pub., 1995.

Rodgers, Bill. *The Complete Idiot's Guide to Jogging and Running*. New York: Alpha Books, 1998.

Runner's World Magazine.

Runner's World Magazine. Runner's World: Training Diary.

Shape Magazine.

Smith, Kathy. *Country Crossroads Audio Workout: Walkfit With Kathy Smith*. New York: Time Warner Audio Books, 1997.

——. *Kathy Smith's Walkfit for a Better Body*. New York: Warner Books, 1994.

——. *Kathy Smith Walkfit: Walking Easy*. New York: Time Warner Audio Books, 1997.

————. *Pump Up the Pace: Walkfit with Kathy Smith* (audio cassette). New York: Time Warner Audio Books, 1997.

Swimming World Magazine.

Vedral, Joyce L., Ph.D. *Weight Training Made Easy: Transform Your Body in Four Simple Steps.*, Warner Books, 1997.

Verna, Chris. *The Complete Idiot's Guide to Healthy Stretching.* New York: Alpha Books, 1998.

Walking Magazine.

Weight Watchers. *Weight Watchers Walk!: New Fun Fitness Walking Workouts!* New York: Simon & Schuster (Audio), 1995.

Westcott, Wayne L. *Building Strength and Stamina: New Nautilus Training for Total Fitness.* Champaign, IL: Human Kinetics Pub., 1996.

SHAPING UP YOUR DIET

Here are some of the most delicious resources for healthy recipes as well as a few books to help you keep track of your eating.

Baggett, Nancy and Ruth Glick. *100% Pleasure.* Emmans, PA: Rodale Books, 1994.

Bellerson, Karen J. *The Complete and Up-to-date Fat Book.* Garden City Park, NY: Avery Publishing Group, 1997.

Cooking Light Magazine.

Cortopassi, Joan and Annette Cain. *Fat Chance, Your Best Chance for Permanent Weight Loss.* Stockton, CA: Alden Books, 1996.

Duyff, Roberta Larson. *The American Dietetic Association's Complete Food & Nutrition Guide.* Minnetonka, MN: Chronimed Publishing, 1996.

Eating Well Magazine.

Fitzpatrick, Nancy J. *Cooking Light Cookbook.* Birmingham, AL: Oxmoor House, Inc., 1995.

Fletcher, Anne. *Eating Thin For Life.* Shelburne, VT: Chapters Publishing Ltd., 1997.

Franz, Marion J. *Exchange for All Occasions.* Minnetonka, MN: Chronimed Pub., 1997.

Franz, Marion J. *Fast Food Facts.* Minnetonka, MN: Chronimed Pub., 1997.

Frederick, Sue. *The Delicious! Collection: Simple Recipes for Healthy Living.* Boulder, CO: New Hope Communications, 1992.

Pennington, Jean. *Bowes & Church's Food Values of Portions Commonly Used.* Philadelphia: J.B. Lippincott Co, 1997.

Rosensweig, Linda. *New Vegetarian Cuisine.* Emmans, PA: Rodale Press, 1993.

Rosso, Julee. *Great Good Food.* Crown Pub, 1993.

Sax, Richard and Marie Simmons. *Lighter, Quicker, Better.* William Morrow & Company, 1995.

Tufts University Diet and Nutrition Letter.

Veggie Life Magazine.

SHAPING UP YOUR ATTITUDE

If you want a little more to help you with your attitude toward shaping up, give any of the following books a try.

Beattie, Melody. *Codependent No More.* San Francisco: Hazeldon/Harper Collins, 1996.

Bloomfield, Dr. Harold H. and Dr. Robert K. Cooper. *The Power of 5.* Emmans, PA: Rodale Books, 1995.

Covey, Stephen. *First Things First.* New York: Simon & Schuster, 1994.

———. *The Seven Habits of Highly Effective People.* GK Hall, 1997.

Estrich, Susan. *Making the Case for Yourself: A Diet Book for Smart Women.* New York: Riverhead Books, 1999.

Evans, William. *Your Pound Shedding Biomarkers.* Fireside, 1992.

Fletcher, Anne. *Thin for Life.* Chapters Pub. Ltd., 1995.

Goor, Dr. Ron and Nancy. *Choose to Lose.* Boston: Houghton Mifflin Co., 1995.

———. *Eater's Choice.* Boston: Houghton Mifflin Co., 1995.

Hay, Louise L. *You Can Heal Your Life.* Carson, CA: Hayhouse, Inc., 1994.

Jordan, Kim. *The Undiet.* Peanut Butter Pub., 1997.

McQuillan, Susan with Dr. Edward Saltzman. *The Complete Idiot's Guide to Losing Weight.* New York: Alpha Books, 1998.

Nelson, Miriam E. *Strong Women Stay Slim.* New York: Bantam Books 1998.

Ornish, Dean. *Eat More, Weigh Less.* New York: Harper Collins, 1997.

Piscatella, Joseph C. *Controlling Your Fat Tooth.* New York: Workman Publishing Co., Inc., 1991.

Prevention Magazine, Emmans, PA: Rodale Press.

Sheehan, George. *Personal Best.* Emmans, PA: Rodale Press.

Waterhouse, Debra. *Why Women Need Chocolate.* New York: Hyperion, 1995.

Winfrey, Oprah and Bob Greene. *Make the Connection.* New York: Hyperion, 1996.

The Weight Control Digest.

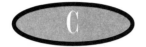

If You Don't Know What It Means/Does, Look Here

DEFINITIONS

aerobic   In the presence of oxygen.

aerobic training   Continuous movement of the larger muscle groups of the body to increase their need for oxygen.

anaerobic training   Also called interval training, this training goes beyond the aerobic state to a threshold beyond which the body cannot supply enough oxygen. This training should only be done in short bursts.

caloric deficit   A loss of energy created when your food energy (calories) is smaller than the total energy (calories) you use, resulting in weight loss.

calorie   A unit of energy used to express the heat output of an organism and the fuel value of food.

cool-down   The gradual tapering off of activity to bring your body back to normal circulation patterns. It should last three to five minutes, minimum.

cross-training Doing a variety of different exercises in your fitness routine and thereby working different muscle groups.

duration Length of time you exercise.

endorphins Natural chemical messengers released by the brain during vigorous exercise, producing feelings of euphoria.

fiber Also referred to as bulk or roughage, it is an indigestible material in human food that stimulates the intestine to peristalsis. The recommended daily intake of fiber is 25 to 30 grams.

flexibility training Also called stretching, this training is an important part of your exercise program. Do stretches only after your muscles are warmed up. Flexibility training will increase your range of motion and circulation and decrease risk of injury and muscle soreness/stiffness.

frequency Number of times you exercise within a week.

intensity Level of exertion while exercising (for example, moderate to hard).

interval training While doing aerobic exercise, you add intervals of speed or intensity to your normal pace (for example, wind sprints). You can become fitter faster with interval training.

isometric exercises These exercises cause tension in a stationary position with no motion of the body limbs (for example, a wall sit).

maximum heart rate The point at which your heart is beating at its maximum level, it can no longer increase its pumping.

metabolism The chemical changes in living cells by which energy is provided for vital processes and activities, such as lean mass energy requirements, digestion, exercise, and daily activities.

repetition (rep) The number of times you repeat an exercise.

resistance   Force applied to the muscle being worked. Forms of resistance include your body, free weights/dumbbells, machines, and elastic/rubber tubing.

resistance band   A strip of rubber (usually 3 to 4 feet long), which is used for strength training (for example, Dynaband or elastic tubing).

resting heart rate   The rate at which your heart beats when you are resting.

set   The number of times you decide to repeat an exercise without a pause.

set point   The constant weight that your body has a tendency to remain at. Lack of exercise, high-fat foods, overeating, and not eating enough (starvation) can raise your body's set point.

stability ball (Swiss ball)   First used to rehabilitate orthopedic and neurological injuries, the stability ball is now popular in the fitness industry and is an excellent tool for improving strength, balance, and coordination.

strength training   Also called resistance training or weightlifting, this type of exercise forces muscles to work hard by introducing resistance to their movement. You can do this with machines, free weights, elastic tubing, or the weight of your own body.

target heart rate   A safe and efficient level of exertion (usually a range such as 65 to 80 percent of your maximum heart rate) where you may be breathing hard, but you can speak easily.

warm up   Starting an aerobic activity gradually to prepare your body for more vigorous exercise. Use your large muscle groups and warm up for at least three to five minutes before increasing intensity.

whole grain   An unprocessed, complex carbohydrate that contains fiber, vitamins, and minerals (for example, brown rice, whole wheat, rye, oat, barley, whole grain cereals). At least half of your breads/cereals/grains servings should be whole grains.

yoga   An eastern mind-body-spirit discipline that involves breathing, balancing, bending, and relaxing. Practicing yoga will make you feel stronger, more balanced and flexible, and more centered. There are a variety of yoga teachings.

NUMBERS/CHARTS

This Amount	Equals This Number of Calories
1 pound of fat	3500 calories
1 gram of carbohydrate	4 calories
1 gram of protein	4 calories
1 gram of fat	9 calories
1 gram of alcohol	7 calories

To track the amount of sugar in processed foods, use this calculation:

1. One teaspoon of sugar equals four grams.

2. The total grams of sugar in a serving divided by four grams per teaspoon equals the number of teaspoons of sugar per serving.

3. The recommended refined sugar intake is 8 to 15 teaspoons per day.

Here's the amount of fat grams you should budget for each day:

- Women are allowed 27 to 44 grams per day.
- Men are allowed 44 to 62 grams per day.

Calculating Resting Heart Rate

You can get a good estimate of your resting heart rate if you count your pulse before getting out of bed in the morning. Lay back and relax, and find your pulse (at your wrist or neck). Count the number of beats for one full minute. Do this for three days and take the average of the days to get your resting heart rate:

Resting heart rate Day 1: _____

Resting heart rate Day 2: _____

Resting heart rate Day 3: _____

Total of all days: _____

Total divided by 3: _____

The final number is your resting heart rate.

Calculating Target Heart Rate Zone

While you do aerobic exercise, your heart rate should remain in a zone that is safe and effective for your age and level of fitness. Your target heart rate zone represents this zone, which is a range between 65 and 80 percent of your maximum heart rate. Target heart rate zones are individual and will vary from person to person. To determine your individual zone, do the following steps:

1. Subtract your age from 220: _____

2. Enter the number from line 1 here: _____. This is your maximum heart rate.

3. Enter your resting heart rate (which you figured out in the preceding section) here: _____

4. Subtract line 3 from line 2: _____

5. Multiply line 4 by .65: _____

6. Multiply line 4 by .85: _____

7. Add line 3 to line 5: _____. This is the lower end of your target zone, per minute.

8. Add line 3 to line 6: _____.

9. Divide line 7 by six: _____. This is the lower end of your target zone, per 10-second interval.

10. Divide line 8 by six: _____. This is the upper end of your target zone, per 10-second interval.

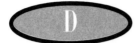

It's Time for Your Reward

Once You've Done This...	Reward Yourself
Scheduled your exercise time	Give yourself a pat on the back
Completed your health screen	Buy a bouquet of flowers
Planned your day of rest	Get a massage
Bought your sneakers (for each activity)	Get a pedicure
Selected your aerobic activities	Listen to your favorite music
Figured out your resting heart rate	Take a nap
Calculated your target heart rate	Enjoy a night out
Taken your measurements	Get a new belt
Made your own dumbbells	Enjoy a workout in nature
Set your fitness goals	Buy a new journal

Where to Find What You're Looking For

Now you can do these tasks, too!

The Lazy Way

Starting to think there are a few more of life's little tasks that you've been putting off? Don't worry—we've got you covered. Take a look at all of *The Lazy Way* books available. Just imagine—you can do almost anything *The Lazy Way!*

Handle Your Money The Lazy Way
By Sarah Young Fisher and Carol Turkington
0-02-862632-X

Build Your Financial Future The Lazy Way
By Terry Meany
0-02-862648-6

Cut Your Spending The Lazy Way
By Leslie Haggin
0-02-863002-5

Have Fun with Your Kids The Lazy Way
By Marilee Lebon
0-02-863166-8

Keep Your Kids Busy The Lazy Way
By Barbara Nielsen and Patrick Wallace
0-02-863013-0

Feed Your Kids Right The Lazy Way
By Virginia Van Vynckt
0-02-863001-7

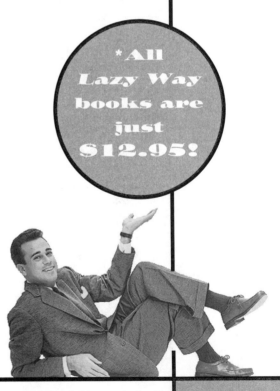

*All Lazy Way books are just $12.95!

additional titles on the back!